Reclaim Your Energy and Feel Normal Again!

Fixing the Root Cause

of Your Fatigue

with Natural Treatments

By Dr. Carri Drzyzga, DC, ND

The Functional Medicine Doc

With a foreword by

Dr. Fraser Smith, BA, ND

Functional Medicine Publishing

Reclaim Your Energy and Feel Normal Again! Fixing the Root Cause of Your Fatigue with Natural Treatments
Functional Medicine Publishing
2543 St. Joseph Blvd.
Orleans, Ontario, K1C 1G2
Canada

ISBN: 978-1500169961

Cover design by Jim Saurbaugh, JS Graphic Design
Interior graphs by Reece Montgomery, Business Book Productions

In memory of my father

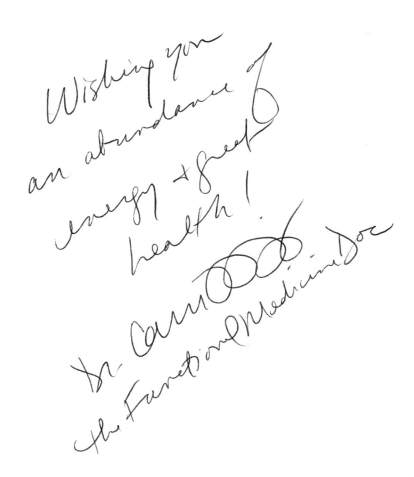

Wishing you an abundance of energy + great health!

Dr. Cann
the Functional Medicine Doc

*"Discovery is seeing
what everybody else has seen,
and thinking
what nobody else has thought."*

—Albert Szent-Györgyi, MD, PhD
Nobel Prize winner for discovering vitamin C

Contents

Foreword.. v
Acknowledgements ix

Part 1
The Hidden, Underlying Causes of Fatigue

Chapter 1—What Is Functional Medicine? 3
  A Personalized, Cause-of-Symptom Approach to Health Care 4
  A Distinction between Natural Medicine and Functional Medicine 6
  Real Stories from Real Women with Fatigue.................................8
  The Eight Leading Causes ("Fatigue Factors") of Fatigue 9

Chapter 2—Fatigue Factor #1: Anemia..11
  Symptoms... 11
  Testing 11
  Treatment.. 12

Chapter 3—Fatigue Factor #2: Thyroid Problems..........................15
  Symptoms... 15
  Testing 16
    Is Your Hypothyroidism Actually Hashimoto's Thyroiditis? 17
    Min's Fatigue Journey—My Eyes Were Always at Half-Mast........ 18
  Treatment.. 29

Chapter 4—Fatigue Factor #3: Cortisol Imbalance 33
  Symptoms... 33
  Testing 35
  Treatment.. 37

Chapter 5—Fatigue Factor #4: Blood Sugar Imbalance...................39
  Symptoms... 39
  Testing 40
    The HbA1C Test 40

What's Your A1C? 40
Treatment 42
You May Be Toxic..42

Chapter 6—Fatigue Factor #5: Nutrient Deficiencies 45
Vitamin B12 Deficiency 45
    Symptoms 45
    Testing 46
    Treatment..47
Vitamin D Deficiency..48
    Symptoms 48
    Jocelyne's Fatigue Journey—Listen to Your Gut Feeling; It's
    Always Right..50
    Testing 62
    Treatment..62
Magnesium Deficiency 62
    Symptoms 62
    Testing 64
    Treatment..65
Iron Deficiency..65
    Symptoms 65
    Testing 66
    Treatment..66
How Do I Know If My Supplements Are Working? Try the Vinegar
Test! 68
Are Acid Blockers Robbing You of Nutrients? Beware of PPIs! 70
    PPI Research (a partial list) 71
    PPIs and Nutrient Deficiencies..72
    Rebound Acidity 73
    How to Safely Get Off Your PPI 73

Chapter 7—Fatigue Factor #6: Chronic Infections 75
Symptoms 75
Testing 77
    Stool Testing 79
    Breath Testing 80
    Ever Wondered if You Really Have IBS or Not? 80
Treatment 81

**Chapter 8—Fatigue Factor #7: Hidden Food Allergies & Sensitivities
....83**
Allergies versus Sensitivities 83
Food Allergies..82
    Symptoms 82
    Testing 82

Food Sensitivities 83
    Symptoms 83
    Testing 84
Treatment for Food Allergies and Sensitivities 85
    The Most Common Food Sensitivities 85
    The Elimination Diet 86

Chapter 9—Fatigue Factor #8: Brain Chemical Imbalance 89
Serotonin 89
    Symptoms 89
Dopamine 90
    Symptoms 90
Testing Serotonin and Dopamine 91
    Brain Balancing—MTO Testing 91
Treatment for Serotonin and Dopamine 91
    Brain Balancing—MTO 91
    Eat Protein 92
    My Fatigue Journey—I Didn't Think It Would Ever Happen to ME! 94

Part 2
Build Your Foundation for *Lasting* Energy

Chapter 10—Energize Your Lifestyle 105
Diet—Let Your Food Be Your Medicine 107
    The Paleo Diet 108
    Blood Sugar and the Paleo Diet 112
    Liz's Fatigue Journey—Now I Actually Feel BETTER Than My Old
    Self!!! 113
    Chronic Low-Grade Inflammation—How It Relates to Fatigue and
    Your Diet 120
Diet—Drink & Hydration 122
    A Solution for Incontinence 122
    Water 123
    Alcohol 124
    Caffeine 125

Chapter 11—Exercise to Enjoy Abundant Energy 127
Exercise and Metabolism 127
    Could You Have a Mitochondrial Imbalance? 128
Beautiful Benefits of Exercise 128

Chapter 12—Sensational Sleep 131
Identify Sleep Disturbers 131

Blood Sugar..131
Cortisol...131
Melatonin...131
Sleep "Hygiene"..133
Good Night, Light!...133
A Restful Routine..134
Marvelous Mattresses...135
Still More Slumber Secrets...135
Anne's Fatigue Journey—Fatigue So Bad That She Slept through a Two-Week Vacation..136

Chapter 13—Vitamin R—Rest, Relaxation, Recreation! 143
Stress Management—Body Chemistry Effects and Solutions 143
Deep Breathing...144
Meditation..145
Two Meditation Samples..145
Yoga..147
Journaling..147
Boxing 148

Chapter 14—You Can Feel Normal Again...Starting Now! 151

Reclaim Your Energy and Feel Normal Again! **Checklist...............155**
Resources 161
Special Bonus 167
Bibliography...169
About the Author..175

Foreword

With the publication of this book, *Reclaim Your Energy and Feel Normal Again! Fixing the Root Cause of Your Fatigue with Natural Treatments*, Dr. Carri Drzyzga has provided patients an invaluable resource for elevating their level of health.

Dr. Drzyzga is in a great position to share this healing advice, having solid practical experience helping patients with fatigue and poor overall health, and having earned professional doctorates in both chiropractic and naturopathic medicine. From this vantage point, she is able to bring some of the very best practices to bear on the issue of fatigue.

It is a mark of an expert that they are able to take a complex subject and explain it in a simple and straightforward manner. Dr. Drzyzga does just that with an accessible writing style and a great structure to her book. Fatigue is prevalent, but the root cause for many patients is unclear. If they are lucky, a rapid medical diagnosis or a change in lifestyle might be the very thing they need. But, for many, the underlying cause of their fatigue and an increasingly poor level of health are unclear.

The conventional care/standard system of medical care that North Americans enjoy addresses many needs for many people and has resulted in spectacular successes in both primary care and tertiary care, such as organ transplants and emergency surgery. However, this system is at its strongest when dealing with discrete lesions or breakdown points in the body, such as a blot clot in a vein, or a tumor on the lung. When patients seek answers to chronic, multifaceted issues such as fatigue, they often find the health care system frustrating, in spite of everyone's best intentions.

The functional medicine approach advocated by Dr. Drzyzga here goes right to the heart of the issues that can contribute to fatigue and ill health. In the first part of this book, a close examination of the nature of fatigue and its causes is laid out in chapters that address major issues, such as hormonal imbalances/deficiency, allergy, nutritional deficiency, and chronic infections. For each of these topics, there is a description of the symptoms and signs, the tests to uncover the causes, and the most common treatment. This is woven together with clinical and case examples that make the topic real and pertinent for the reader.

The second part of the book gives the reader a lasting gift—clear-cut instructions on how to lay the foundation for long-term good health. The key is to take specific actions to address the determining factors of health. This is followed by useful tools at the end of the book to support recovery and health maintenance.

While this book does indeed teach some complex issues in a straightforward way, it is at the same time rich in information, and Dr. Drzyzga's expertise shines through. These important precepts are taught with skill, compassion, respect for all approaches, and interventions that a patient might need, and taken together can offer the reader who suffers from fatigue new hope. The best health care combines intelligent self-help along with expert guidance. This book is really an invitation to the reader to work with a functional medicine/natural medicine professional and other members of the care team to explore the issues that could very well be a turning point in their recovery.

—Dr. Fraser Smith, BA, ND

Associate Professor, National University of Health Sciences

Assistant Dean, Naturopathic Medicine, National University of Health Sciences

Author of *An Introduction to Principles & Practices of Naturopathic Medicine* and *Keep Your Brain Young: A Health and Diet Program for Your Brain*

Coauthor of *The pH Balance Health and Diet Guide for GERD, IBS and IBD*

Acknowledgements

I owe a debt of immense gratitude to my mentors: Dr. Alex Vasquez, DC, ND, DO; Dr. Datis Kharrazian, DHSc, DC, MS; Dr. Tom O'Bryan, DC, CCN, DACBN; Dr. Daniel Kalish, DC; Dr. Mehmet Oz, MD; Dr. Mark Hyman, MD; and Dr. Jeffery Bland, PhD, FACN, CNS. You are all trailblazers and have had a major impact on my career. For that I will be forever grateful.

A special thank you to Dr. David Lescheid, PhD, ND for introducing me to naturopathic medicine.

My sincere appreciation to Dr. Fraser Smith, BA, ND for writing the foreword.

To Anne, Jocelyne, Liz, and Min: I cannot thank you enough for having the courage and generosity to share your stories in this book. You are a group of amazing and strong women.

Thank you to all my patients for your continued support throughout the years. It's an honor and a privilege to serve you.

To my dream team: Susan and Magda, you are awesome assistants. Thank you for taking such great care of our patients and for everything you do at the office to keep it running smoothly. The amazing growth of my practice would not be possible without your incredible support.

To my business coach, Jim Palmer: Thank you for all your wisdom, encouraging words, and tough love. Without you this book would still only be a pipe dream.

A big thank you to my wonderful editor, Tammy Barley; and to Jim Saurbaugh and Reece Montgomery for their cover design and interior artistry.

To Benoit, my husband, my partner, my best friend, and soul mate: You continue to be the greatest blessing in my life.

Thank you to Mom, Dad, my family, and friends for all your support. Special thanks to my bestest friend and fellow Leo (you know who you are!).

Part 1

The Hidden, Underlying Causes
of Fatigue

Chapter 1

What Is Functional Medicine?

Functional medicine is a new and emerging field of healthcare. It's a subspecialty within the much broader field of natural medicine.

Thousands of women today suffer with fatigue, yet are commonly told by their doctors, "All your test results are normal," except that their fatigue continues to get worse. Women are even told, "You just need a vacation," or "You're depressed," or "It's all in your head," or other such nonsense. Eventually these women feel that their doctors don't know what to do with them anymore, and they get tired of being offered Band-Aid solutions like antidepressants and sleeping pills.

Fatigue is one of the most common complaints in doctors' offices, yet it is one of the most poorly managed and misunderstood illnesses. Until now.

While medical doctors typically address patients' symptoms, functional medicine is about finding and fixing the underlying cause of those symptoms, so patients experience real and lasting results.

Functional medicine practitioners pinpoint the root, underlying cause of fatigue and then work with their patients to fix it, using treatments that are natural, safe, and proven effective.

This approach enables women to feel normal again, get their health and energy back, and become able to enjoy life to the fullest.

Find the cause. Fix the cause. Feel normal again! That's functional medicine in a nutshell.

A Personalized, Cause-of-Symptom Approach to Health Care

Everything in your body is connected. When medical doctors prescribe a medication to correct one complaint, seemingly unrelated systems in the body are often affected adversely by the medication. Functional medicine doctors understand this, so we tend to think "outside the box," not only in how we diagnose, but also in how we heal.

We also look at each and every patient as unique, even if they all suffer with the same problem: fatigue.

That means every patient gets a personalized approach to care, and a personalized approach to treatment. There's no "one-size-fits-all" approach—that doesn't work with T-shirts, and it certainly doesn't work with fatigue!

Maybe you're not only troubled with your fatigue. Your foggy brain may be worrying you too. You can't concentrate very well, and your memory is slowly getting worse. You walk into a room and forget why you went there in the first place. You forget phone numbers and names. You make more and more lists because your brain isn't as sharp as it used to be.

Perhaps you've even tried some supplements but they didn't work for you. Or you're hesitant about trying them because you're not a professional and you don't want to make matters worse. And, you certainly don't want to waste your money taking vitamins that you may not even need in the first place.

One thing you do know is this: If you never find the underlying cause of your fatigue, you will probably never get better. And getting better is your only option.

With fatigue, the standard medical approach consists of testing for 1) anemia, and 2) low thyroid, which is an important first step. Anemia and low thyroid can cause fatigue, and *always* should be tested first. The problem is, the majority of the time these tests are normal, and if you're otherwise healthy, then your doctor doesn't know what to do next beyond offering you an antidepressant.

Functional medicine doctors look at the whole body, not just one area, *because* everything in your body is connected. We want to hear about everything that's going on with your health—all your complaints, all at once—so we can piece those connections together.

That is usually what takes place during a first visit with a functional medicine doctor. This is where the detective work starts. A thorough history from a patient will often reveal the clues needed to crack your case wide open. A functional medicine doctor will then look over all the tests that your family doctor and specialists have already run. That leads to even more clues, then further testing, to find the underlying cause of your fatigue.

That is also how this book begins—by analyzing the most likely underlying cause(s) of your fatigue.

After the functional medicine doctor finds the cause(s) of a patient's fatigue, then the patient's treatment plan is put together—an actual plan designed specifically for her. It's very much a team approach. The functional medicine doctor and patient work together, as mutual allies.

That is how this book continues, albeit without the benefit of an individually tailored plan—by providing a plan of solutions proven to build a foundation of lasting energy for most patients.

Functional medicine is a patient-centered approach, not a disease-centered approach. Patient-centered means we treat *you*. We find what is out of balance with you, and then treat you for that.

Treatment may include vitamins, herbs, diet changes, and the like, then we retest to ensure all normal function and energy levels are returning.

A Distinction between Natural Medicine and Functional Medicine

To illustrate the distinction between natural and functional medicine approaches to treating fatigue, here's an example.

Sometimes fatigue is caused by lack of sleep. Either you have a hard time falling asleep or you wake up in the middle of the night—a very obvious reason why you would have fatigue, right?

Many *natural health* practitioners would approach this and say, "Take melatonin."

So, instead of prescribing a sleeping pill, they prescribe you the "natural" equivalent, which is melatonin. This is called "green allopathy"—directly substituting a natural supplement instead of a medication. It sometimes works, but often it doesn't. It's "natural," but it's not actually treating the underlying cause of the sleeping problem.

It's not *functional medicine*.

Here's what goes on inside my mind as a functional medicine doctor.

First, I understand how melatonin is made in the body (melatonin is made from serotonin, which is made from 5-HTP, which is made from tryptophan—this is the basic chemistry of it), and also what it does in the body (this is why you shouldn't get advice from health food store employees—they don't have this level of training). And then I test for melatonin deficiency.

If there is no melatonin deficiency, taking melatonin supplements obviously won't work. You would just waste your time and money.

If there is a melatonin deficiency, then I find out why—what is *causing* the melatonin to be low? I don't just give a melatonin supplement.

If the "why" is never fixed and the underlying cause of the deficiency is never found, that means you would have to take the melatonin supplements for the rest of your life! That's not what you want! And, it's not what I want for you either.

So now I figure out the "why" and look for the cause: Is there not enough of the building-block nutrients to make melatonin? Is melatonin getting used up faster than it can be produced? Is something blocking melatonin production, like iron deficiency? Or, protein deficiency? Is there a serotonin deficiency?

If the melatonin test is normal, then I keep looking for the underlying cause of the insomnia.

Here are the questions that go through my head next. Is cortisol too high at night? Is the blood sugar dropping during the night sooner than it should? Is there a blockage in an acupuncture channel? Is there a blockage in the liver detox pathways allowing caffeine to stay in the bloodstream too long? Is magnesium deficient? Is there a hidden food allergy? And on, and on, always searching out the underlying cause (in this case, the underlying cause of the insomnia that is creating the fatigue).

I know that may be a little technical and "doctor-y," so I certainly don't expect you to understand all of it. But, I do want you to see that functional medicine is *not* Band-Aid medicine that treats only surface symptoms.

In functional medicine, we always seek to find the cause and fix the cause naturally.

Always.

That's why functional medicine works when other approaches don't. That is why functional medicine is an exciting, emerging field of healthcare.

Real Stories from Real Women with Fatigue

I want you to see how functional medicine actually works in real life and why it works so well. So I've included five real cases from my private practice—four of my patients' fatigue stories as well as my personal fatigue story. We all had fatigue, but all for different reasons, so we all received different treatments.

Ironically, my fatigue was the hardest of the five to treat! You know what they say: live and learn. I guess I took that literally! That's why I'm so dedicated to helping other women who have fatigue—so they can get their lives back.

You'll get to see our stories, our struggles, and our triumphs. My hope is that you will be encouraged to have hope and to get that same help and relief for yourself.

Sometimes it may feel like there's no answer, but I want you to know you should have *a lot* of hope. Note that I said, "We all *had* fatigue." Today all five of us live fatigue-free, with the normal levels of energy we were designed to have.

I won't kid you—sometimes finding the underlying cause of fatigue can feel like finding a needle in a haystack. But the underlying cause *is* there, just waiting to be discovered.

The Eight Leading Causes ("Fatigue Factors") of Fatigue

I have discovered fourteen causes for fatigue. This book delves into the first eight on my list, since they apply to the majority of women suffering with fatigue.

Here they are for you. I call this is my Basic Fatigue List.

1. Anemia
2. Thyroid Problems
3. Cortisol Imbalance
4. Blood Sugar Imbalance
5. Nutrient Deficiencies
6. Chronic Infections
7. Hidden Food Allergies & Sensitivities
8. Brain Imbalance

Besides "fatigue factors" #1 and #2, the rest of this list is in no particular order of importance. A good history can help point the right direction to go next.

Also, it's rare that just one factor on this list is causing the fatigue. Most of the time, there are multiple issues that need to be addressed on the list—usually three or four (or more) need to be addressed. Again, there's no cookie-cutter protocol to treat fatigue.

Note: You can get a free copy of my Expanded List, which details the six additional fatigue factors not included in my Basic Fatigue List. They are especially for more complicated fatigue cases—like when fatigue seems to be genetic, or when you've already "tried everything else." Go to the Special Bonus section at the end of this book to learn how to claim your free copy.

So it's wise to work with a functional medicine doctor, especially one who specializes in fatigue, to guide you in the right direction for your case. Otherwise, you'll most likely waste a lot of time and money.

Now, let's explore these eight leading causes of fatigue.

Chapter 2

Fatigue Factor #1: Anemia

Symptoms

When you have fatigue, anemia should *always* be checked first.

Anemia means your red blood cells are low or your hemoglobin is low. In addition to fatigue, you might also experience:

> ➤ rapid heartbeat (more so when exercising)
> ➤ headache and/or shortness of breath (more so when exercising)
> ➤ dizziness
> ➤ difficulty concentrating
> ➤ paleness of skin
> ➤ cold hands and feet
> ➤ leg cramps
> ➤ chest pain
> ➤ insomnia

Anemia is one of the most common signs of Celiac disease (and it's often the first sign!).

Testing

Medical doctors routinely check this with a CBC (complete blood count). This test measures your red blood cells, white blood cells, hemoglobin, and other things.

In the majority of fatigue patients, the test results come back as normal.

However, when it is abnormal and there is anemia present, the next step is to figure out *why* the anemia is there in the first place.

Seems logical, I know, except most doctors don't do it. They jump right into prescribing iron supplements (or B12 injections). But the goal should always be to find the cause. In this case, find the cause of the anemia.

Treatment

If testing shows you have anemia, this is what should be explored next. I will use iron deficiency anemia in this example, but the following thought process should also take place for B12 deficiency anemia.

➢ Are you not getting enough iron from your diet?

➢ Is iron not being absorbed properly? (H. pylori infection in the stomach is a common reason for this, as is silent Celiac disease.)

➢ Is iron being used up faster than it's getting put in? (Bacterial overgrowth in the small intestine, or SIBO, is a common reason for this. The bacteria feed on the iron and steal it from you.)

➢ Are you leaking iron from somewhere? (A bleeding ulcer or a bleeding polyp will cause you to lose blood and iron. This blood loss is usually not visible in your stool.)

Anemia can be the first and only warning sign of something seriously wrong, like cancer or silent Celiac disease. Anemia should always been taken seriously and investigated fully. Period.

In the case of iron deficiency, this includes scoping the entire digestive tract for bleeding, and being tested for silent Celiac disease and H. pylori infection. If your doctor has not done these things, or recommended that you do these things, you need to find a new doctor.

Lastly, if any of your family members have anemia too, you should automatically be checked for Celiac disease, non-Celiac gluten sensitivity, and pernicious anemia. These are all more common than you might think, and usually go undiagnosed.

In fact, you may be the first member of your family to be properly diagnosed for the cause of your anemia, and the underlying cause of your fatigue.

Chapter 3

Fatigue Factor #2: Thyroid Problems

Symptoms

After checking for anemia, the thyroid should *always* be checked next as a possible underlying cause of your fatigue.

Fatigue is a common symptom of low thyroid, or hypothyroidism. Other low-thyroid symptoms can include:

- poor circulation
- sensitivity to cold
- dry skin
- thinning hair
- outer third of eyebrows thin or bald
- poor memory
- depression
- constipation
- weight gain
- high cholesterol

Low thyroid function, like anemia, is not at all uncommon. Here is a list of the TSH (thyroid stimulating hormone) levels for the fatigue patients featured in this book:

TSH Levels Ideally 0.3-2.0	
Anne	1.84
Jocelyne	2.33
Liz	2.64
Min	2.96
Dr. Carri	7.15

As you see, four out of five patients had thyroid levels above ideal, meaning their thyroid was getting weak. Low thyroid function is common even for patients already on thyroid medications, which means their medication dosage still needs to be adjusted further.

By the way, know that what is considered "normal" levels and what is considered to be "ideal" levels varies greatly. Your doctor is probably using "normal" levels. I use "ideal" levels for optimal health.

Testing

Doctors test thyroid function with a TSH blood test.

Unfortunately, most doctors are still using the older guidelines when it comes to interpreting this test, so many women's thyroid problems are being missed.

It's better to use the guidelines recommended by the American Academy of Clinical Endocrinologists. They consider a TSH of 0.3-3.0 as normal. A TSH above 2.0 is the start of a thyroid problem, and a TSH above 3.0 is considered low thyroid.

Basically, the higher your TSH number gets, the weaker your thyroid is getting.

A TSH above 2.0 should be further investigated with thyroid antibody testing— anti-thyroperoxidase (anti-TPO) antibodies and anti-thyroglobulin (anti-TG) antibodies. These are simple blood tests. When antibodies are present, the case goes from a simple low thyroid to a more complicated immune system problem called Hashimoto's Thyroiditis, which is still fixable.

> Whenever you get any testing done, make sure to get a copy for your own records so you can see what your numbers are.
>
> (Some patients are reluctant to do this. Don't be! They're *your* records, and you're entitled to a copy for yourself! No one will care more about the meaning of your test results than you.)

(Thyroid antibodies are like chemical bullets that your body makes and aims straight at your thyroid, slowly destroying it.)

Is Your Hypothyroidism Actually Hashimoto's Thyroiditis?

If thyroid problems run in your family, or if your medical doctor has a difficult time figuring out what dose of thyroid medication is right for you, there is a strong possibility that you actually have Hashimoto's Thyroiditis and not regular hypothyroidism. Anti-TPO and anti-TG antibody testing will confirm if this is true for you.

This was the case with Min. When I did further testing on the five women featured in this book, Min was found to actually have

Hashimoto's Thyroiditis. As soon as we uncovered this, her treatment plan changed dramatically. And Min's fatigue finally started to improve! (Find the cause. Fix the cause. Feel normal again!)

Min's Fatigue Journey— My Eyes Were Always at Half-Mast

Dr. Carri: Hi, Min! Thank you for sitting down with me to share your fatigue story. I know your story will help encourage our readers to have hope that they can have normal energy again. Let's get started.

Tell me about your fatigue. How long did you have it? What other doctors did you see? What other treatments did you try? What was your life like back when you had fatigue?

Min: My fatigue started almost two years ago now. I just didn't have energy. I would go into sweats—I called them "exhaustion sweats." I was totally exhausted, and I would just start to sweat. And then I was very, very tired, so tired that I couldn't get off the couch. My eyes were always at half-mast.

My head felt full, heavy, like there were marbles in it. That's why I was lying down all the time. I couldn't hold my head up. And it felt like someone was sitting on my chest. Most days this is how I lived.

My kids complained that mom didn't do anything except sleep on the couch. That's literally what I did—slept on the couch all winter long.

I finally went to see my family doctor. She ordered blood work and tweaked my thyroid medication. It didn't help. So she tweaked my thyroid medication again. Now I was alternating between two different doses every other day. Try and remember that when you're feeling so tired and your brain's not working! It's awful! And it still didn't help. So I got fed up!

Then she wanted to tweak my medicine once more, and I thought, "No, I can't do it. I'm going to see Dr. Carri!" I've known you for years, and I thought you were my best hope to make me feel better.

So that's how I got to see you. I figured if anyone knew how to fix my problem it would be you.

Dr. Carri: Did your family doctor ever offer anything else? Like antidepressants?

Min: Oh yes! I refused to go on them! I said, "I'm not depressed. I am *not* depressed. I *know* I am not depressed."

Dr. Carri: A lot of family doctors tend to recommend antidepressants for fatigue patients. And the patients know they're not depressed. They say "no" because they know deep down inside that it's not depression; it's something else going on.

Min: She said to me, "Look, your plate is full," and I said, "I know my plate is full. But it should not make me feel so tired that I can't do my daily chores." I finally told my doctor I would try the antidepressants just to appease her, but I never tried them. I just told her they didn't work. I lied!

That's when desperation came. I was disheartened, but not depressed. So when I came to you and dumped on you that day... You know the stress I'm under. I have a disabled son, a daughter who feels she's entitled to the world, and my husband deceased by eight years. It's hard. But I knew I wasn't depressed.

I knew there was something else going on, and that's when you decided to do more blood work to find out what was really going on with me.

Dr. Carri: What other symptoms were you having besides the fatigue? You had mentioned feeling a weight on your chest, the sweats, marbles in your brain—would you call that foggy brain?

Min: Yeah! It's a real fog! You just can't think! You try to think something through, or somebody asks you a question, and I'm thinking to myself, "How do I answer that question?" But I just can't find the answer in my brain. It's there, but I can't find it through the layers of fog. I couldn't find the answers to even simple questions.

And I had gained weight—twenty pounds. My clothes were feeling wretchedly tight. I had to go buy new clothes. That's disheartening!

Dr. Carri: Was there anything about having the fatigue that had you really worried, or angry, or frustrated?

Min: I was pissed! I really was! You figure you go to a doctor and they should help you out. But I know their hands are tied. That's the health care system for you.

Plus I have my two kids to take care of. One is disabled, as you know, and there's no help for him right now, no group home for him in sight, so I have to look after him. I have to stay healthy to do that. I have to stay healthy for him, because there's no one else to take care of him.

Dr. Carri: What were your top three daily frustrations?

Min: I couldn't read. I couldn't keep my eyes open. I couldn't manage a half hour TV show before my eyes were closed. Simple things like that. I couldn't follow a conversation. I still drove, but it was difficult. I worried that I might fall asleep behind the wheel someday.

Dr. Carri: Then we sat down, you and I, and we talked about your thyroid history. How many people in your family have a thyroid problem?

Min: One sister, two nieces, my aunt, my grandmother. Thyroid problems run in my family.

Dr. Carri: So, multiple women in your family with thyroid problems—there's got to be a genetic cause there. That's one thing I want people to understand.

Thyroid problems are common, but when you look into the family tree and see other people having thyroid problems, you need to dig into that thyroid issue deeper and see where it's really coming from. Min, that's one of the things we did for you. I requested your blood work to see what your doctor had tested. And I know your doctor told you all your tests were normal.

I'll look at that same blood work and find issues, because I'm looking to see if your numbers are *ideal* or not, not just are they "in the normal range."

For you we found that your iron was *way* too low. It was obviously low. Your doctor should have seen that. And of course that's a big cause of fatigue right there—low iron. Your B12 was low too. Your vitamin D was low. And your thyroid was still too low, even though you were on your thyroid medication.

So with your basic blood work we found more than one reason why you were having fatigue. And then we delved deeper into the thyroid, because of your family history and because your doctor was having a hard time balancing out your thyroid hormones.

That's another thing I want people to understand. If your doctor has a hard time finding the right dose of thyroid medication for you, that is a big red flag that you probably have Hashimoto's—you probably have an autoimmune thyroid condition going on. And that's what you should be tested for.

That's what we tested you for, Min, and found that you actually have Hashimoto's.

The significance of that means there's a whole other problem going on in your body, with your immune system attacking your thyroid. It's way bigger than just a low thyroid.

Your family doctor has been very gracious about running the tests that I asked for. She really wants you to get better. But like you said, her hands are tied within the health care system.

So, we figured this out, the Hashimoto's, and this is why I wanted your story to be in this book.

A lot of women struggling with fatigue think they have a thyroid problem, but their doctors keep telling them, "No, your tests are normal," but they actually *do* have a thyroid problem.

And a lot of women who are diagnosed with a thyroid problem are still not getting adequate care either, because what they actually have is Hashimoto's, like you. But most doctors never test for that.

To sum up, for your fatigue we found: not enough B12, not enough iron, not enough vitamin D, your thyroid needed more support, and you specifically had Hashimoto's. So we found five reasons why you had fatigue just with that blood work.

Min: That's a lot! And then you had me take supplements and change my diet.

Dr. Carri: Yes, with Hashimoto's there's a big correlation between having gluten sensitivity—even Celiac disease—and Hashimoto's. So one thing I recommended is that you and your family go on a gluten-free diet.

Min: Once I started the gluten-free diet, it was strange—not difficult—just strange not to have a piece of bread or a doughnut like you're used to eating. Now I can feel it within a half hour if I've eaten something that's got gluten in it. I get horrendous abdominal pain and bloating, and I get tired. Gluten is a big sensitivity for me.

After about three months of supplements and the gluten-free diet, I actually felt like a human being again! I had myself back! I thought, "I'm me again!"

So I'm trucking along feeling pretty good, and the next thing I know I'm feeling tired again. There's something wrong. I didn't realize it, but I was forgetting to take my B12! So I started taking it again, and my energy came back.

Dr. Carri: We'd gotten new blood work to see what was changing—what's working, what wasn't working—and I saw that your B12 didn't improve all that much, and that's what you said—you had stopped taking your B12. You just forgot that one.

We also saw that your iron level didn't improve. It was lower, worse than before. Some patients can be really tricky like this. We have to figure out what works best for *you*. Because everybody is unique and different, even with something simple like an iron supplement, we have to figure out what works best for *you*.

I'm certain once we get your iron levels up, you're going to have lots more energy.

Since starting your treatment program, your thyroid has drastically improved. You're still making antibodies, which means your body is still sending chemical bullets at your thyroid, and that's what we're trying to stop, but your thyroid function itself has improved immensely.

Min: I'm still a work in progress.

Dr. Carri: Yes, we're about six months into your case.

Min: And I'm feeling so much better! I'm getting excited about feeling like my old self again!

Dr. Carri: Now that you're feeling better, what are you doing now that you couldn't do before?

Min: I'm walking! I'm reading! I finished a book! I love reading; I've always been an avid reader, so being able to read again is huge. And I started sewing again! I'm working on my piles—getting all that stuff done that's been piling up.

Dr. Carri: Do you have any advice for other women struggling with fatigue?

Min: Oh, I do! If you have a doctor who has told you there is nothing wrong with you, please find someone who can help you, like a naturopath who knows functional medicine. Someone who will help find the cause.

And don't blame yourself! I was doing that—blaming myself for the fatigue. It's not your fault!

I don't know if it's just me or if all women are like that, blame themselves for things that go wrong. It's not your fault.

And another thing. If it's in your family, tell your other family members so they're aware and can get help for themselves. I called everyone in my family and told them this is what's been discovered in me, so get yourself checked too!

Dr. Carri: Yes, everyone in your family should be checked for Hashimoto's, and everyone should be screened for gluten sensitivity and Celiac disease. All your blood relatives should be checked.

When I initially recommended that gluten-free diet, what did you think?

Min: I thought, "No, it can't be that. It can't be. I've been eating this all along and haven't had any digestive problems, aside from a bit of constipation." And now that I look back at my life, it all started at eighteen years old. I had abdominal pains so bad. I remember that now!

Dr. Carri: So it's possible that gluten has been a problem since you were eighteen. Who really knows unless we build a time machine? But it's definitely possible. How old were you when your thyroid problem was diagnosed?

Min: It was after my son was born. I was around forty-three.

Dr. Carri: And that was another point that I wanted to bring up. This happens to a lot of women. They are never well since the birth of their last child. Their body just never recovers. Especially if you end up with a thyroid problem after your last child, 98 percent of the time that's actually an autoimmune thyroid going on—Hashimoto's. Like you, Min.

With autoimmune conditions, we now have testing for these antibodies. It's called predictive antibody testing. Your body will give off these antibodies, or "chemical bullets," for five to ten years before your diagnosis. We can find antibodies in the blood stream now for something like rheumatoid arthritis, but if you never make any changes to your lifestyle, you will most likely end up with a full-blown case of rheumatoid arthritis in due time. You're just a ticking time bomb, within five to ten years. It's a miracle of science that we have this predictive antibody testing now.

So for you, Min, you remember at eighteen years old this terrible abdominal pain. This may have been a slow, smoldering fire in your body. Then twenty-five years later you're diagnosed with a thyroid problem, which has probably been Hashimoto's the whole time. That's textbook.

Min: Yes, and I was going through so much stress at that time too. Stress finding a job. Stress with my son, finding out about his disability—that puts extra stress on a parent. Yes, that was a highly stressful period for me.

Dr. Carri: Stress has a *big* impact on the body. Min, do you have any other advice for our readers? I guess we were talking about the gluten....

Min: Try the gluten-free diet! It's not going to hurt! That's what I told myself. And I also thought, "I'm going to show her this is not going to work! I'll prove to her it's not gluten!" (Laughs.) At least I'm being honest with you! And low and behold, you were right!

Anyway, gluten-free is not as hard as you may think. There are a lot of gluten-free options out there these days.

Dr. Carri: I had that same experience with going gluten-free. I resisted it for years. I convinced myself that it couldn't be gluten, and the diet would be too hard. I had a real mental block on it! And then one day I decided to pull the trigger, and I slowly transitioned over to a gluten-free diet. Then like you, I thought, "Hey, that wasn't too hard. Why didn't I do this years ago? Duh!" (Laughs.)

Going gluten-free is mainly a mental block. A hurdle. Like climbing Mount Everest. People do that every day, just by putting one step in front of another.

Is there anything else you want to add?

Min: *Thank you.* I'm glad to be feeling more like my old self!

Dr. Carri: Thank *you* for sharing your story. I'm glad you're feeling so much better.

Most patients who have already been diagnosed with low thyroid are never even checked for anti-TPO and anti-TG antibodies. So, if you already know you have a low thyroid, the next thing to do is see if you have Hashimoto's Thyroiditis with anti-TPO and anti-TG antibody testing.

Note: Most doctors don't test for antibodies because that does not change their treatment plan, which is to give you thyroid medications for the rest of your life!

So if you ask for these tests and your doctor says no, just keep pushing. Tell them you want to know if you really have Hashimoto's or not.

Hashimoto's will change your treatment plan dramatically from a functional medicine standpoint. In my office, a simple case of low thyroid gets treated radically different than Hashimoto's.

Treatment

In the TSH Levels chart, you can see that my thyroid was very weak, even by medical standards! I was clearly hypothyroid.

TSH Levels Ideally 0.3-2.0	
Anne	1.84
Jocelyne	2.33
Liz	2.64
Min	2.96
Dr. Carri	7.15

But, wouldn't you know it—my family doctor actually said to me, "We don't usually treat this until your TSH gets into double digits."

What?

I wasn't going to wait around for my thyroid to get worse! I only have one, and it has to last me the rest of my life!

That's when I took my case into my own hands and applied all the principles of functional medicine: Find the cause. Fix the cause. Feel normal again!

Unfortunately, when it comes to low thyroid, finding the cause isn't always an easy task. However, there is *always* a reason why the thyroid gets low.

The details behind investigating and fixing low thyroid could fill an entire book, so for now I'll give you the broad brushstrokes.

➢ A high TSH level just tells you one thing—that your thyroid is weak. It gives no indication as to *why* your thyroid is weak. That's why further investigation must take place.

➢ Once weak thyroid has been discovered, the next step should be a full thyroid workup. This includes testing all the thyroid hormones (free T3, free T4, total T3, total T4, and reverse T3), and the antibodies anti-TPO and anti-TG, which I spoke of earlier. Ask your doctor for these tests.

➢ And, from the Basic Fatigue List, fatigue factors #3 Cortisol Imbalance and #4 Blood Sugar Imbalance should also be checked, as they are often at the root of low thyroid.

➢ Fatigue factor #5 Nutrient Deficiencies should be considered too, because many key nutrients are required for thyroid hormone production. These include:
- ✓ iodine
- ✓ selenium
- ✓ zinc
- ✓ copper
- ✓ vitamin A

➢ The other fatigue factors that will commonly cause low thyroid and therefore should be checked include hormonal imbalances (specifically, low progesterone and estrogen surges) and heavy metal toxicity. These fatigue factors are included in my Expanded Fatigue List (to get a free copy of this list, please refer to the Special Bonus section at the end of this book).

If you have Hashimoto's, you would do all of the above to investigate the thyroid, plus investigate the biggest piece of the Hashimoto's puzzle—*your immune system*—because that's what Hashimoto's is—your immune system attacking your thyroid by using chemical bullets.

As with low thyroid, there is no cookie-cutter approach for fixing Hashimoto's. Getting your immune system to "behave" and "play nice" with your thyroid requires a multipronged approach. It's not easy. Again, here are the broad brushstrokes.

(By the way, what I recommend below applies to any and all autoimmune diseases, not just Hashimoto's.)

➢ With all autoimmune diseases, including Hashimoto's, there is usually a low-grade infection somewhere in the body. The infection is part of what is fueling the immune attack. In medical lingo this is termed "molecular mimicry." Use the information from fatigue factor #6 Chronic Infections to help find your hidden infection.

➢ There are key nutrients required to create balance within your immune system. They are known as immunomodulators and include:
  ✓ vitamin D
  ✓ vitamin A
  ✓ essential fatty acids EPA and DHA
  ✓ probiotics
  ✓ lipoic acid
  ✓ N-acetylcysteine
  ✓ superoxide dismutase
  ✓ selenium (this one is specific for Hashimoto's)

➢ Determining which specific arm of your immune system is overacting is no easy task, and is beyond the scope of this book. But, please know that this can be treated with specific herbs.

➢ Gluten sensitivity is a big trigger for many autoimmune diseases, including Hashimoto's. Following a 100 percent gluten-free diet is always advisable.

➢ Fatigue factor #7 Hidden Food Allergies & Sensitivities should always be checked as well. Whenever you eat a food that you are allergic or sensitive to, it creates an upsurge in your immune response. This upsurge usually leads to more chemical bullets aimed at your thyroid. This is not what you want! Eat only the foods you know are your friends—the foods you are not allergic or sensitive to. For more information, see Chapter 8.

➢ Lastly, there is a lot of controversy over whether or not it is safe to use iodine, as a supplement or in kelp preparations, with Hashimoto's. I lead toward the do-not-use-iodine-if-you-have-Hashimoto's camp until more conclusive research is available.

Chapter 4

Fatigue Factor #3: Cortisol Imbalance

Symptoms

Cortisol imbalance is the most common cause of fatigue. I place it third on my list of fatigue factors since anemia and thyroid should always be checked first.

Cortisol is a hormone secreted by the adrenal glands during times of chronic stress. In fact, if your fatigue started six to twelve months after a major stress, then cortisol is likely to blame. Major stress can include death or critical illness of a loved one, separation or divorce, the effects or aftereffects of abuse, loss of employment, surgery, pregnancy, or any other chronic stress.

When you're under chronic stress, your cortisol gets out of balance. Then the domino effect starts, because cortisol impacts twelve different body systems: your immune system, hormones, digestive tract, brain, thyroid, metabolism.... It affects nearly everything!

Then the stress leaves. And life gets back to "normal." Except *you* don't get back to normal. You don't feel normal. You still have fatigue. And you feel like you're falling apart (which you kind of are).

This is because once your cortisol is out of balance, it will continue to be out of balance, like a runaway train. It will create chaos in your body until you're diagnosed and treated properly, until your cortisol is back to normal.

Aside from fatigue, symptoms of cortisol imbalance may include:

➢ not sleeping well
➢ wake up tired, even after a full night's sleep
➢ craving sweet and/or salty foods
➢ feeling run-down
➢ surge of energy in the evening
➢ weight gain around the waist
➢ feeling overwhelmed or unable to cope with stress
➢ get colds and infections easily
➢ low or poor stamina
➢ slow to recover from injury or illness
➢ low blood pressure
➢ difficulty concentrating

Cortisol is normally highest in the morning when you wake up. In fact, this is actually what triggers you to wake up. So if your cortisol is too low in the morning, you will have a hard time getting out of bed. You will want to hit that snooze button over and over again! Basically, you are starting your day tired, even if you did get plenty of sleep.

Cortisol is normally lowest at night for deepest sleep. When cortisol is too high at night, you won't get good, deep sleep and will suffer from sleep deprivation. You can see how that would lead to fatigue.

There are basically three stages of cortisol imbalance: cortisol can be too high all day long, too low all day long, or it can be like a roller coaster throughout your day.

The only way to know what your cortisol is doing is to get tested.

Testing

Cortisol should always be tested with a saliva test, one that includes four saliva samples collected and measured throughout your average, typical day.

If your doctor doesn't offer you a saliva test for cortisol, find one who will. Again, hands down this is the most common cause of fatigue that I see in my practice. And, it's totally fixable.

Here are three real-life examples of cortisol imbalance found using saliva testing:

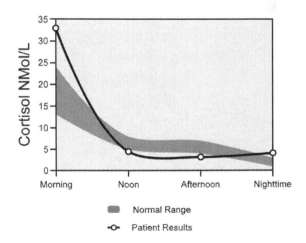

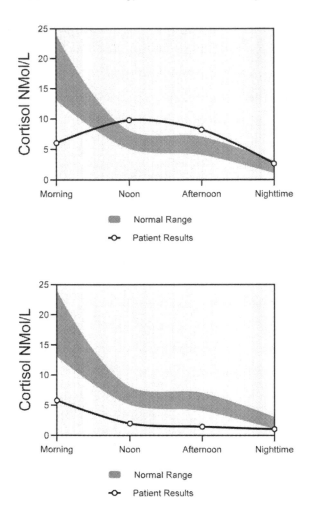

Normal Range

Patient Results

You can clearly see the differences in these test results even though these three patients all had the same problem—fatigue.

Don't rely on your symptoms alone to determine if your cortisol is too high or too low (and neither should your doctor!). Doing so would most likely only lead you on a wild goose chase.

Again, the only way to really know what your cortisol is doing is to get tested with a saliva test, one that requires four saliva samples.

Treatment

Finding out that your cortisol is out of balance is the first step. The next step is to find out why your cortisol is out of balance. There's *always* a reason why the cortisol goes wonky.

Unfortunately, there is no cookie-cutter approach to treating cortisol imbalance. But here are the broad brushstrokes.

➢ Once cortisol is out of balance, it will have a domino effect and create weakness in the intestines. What happens next is usually fatigue factor #6 Hidden Infections and/or fatigue factor #7 Hidden Food Allergies & Sensitivities. Both should be checked because they will compound the stress on your body and create a vicious cycle which continues to fuel the cortisol imbalance. And around and around it goes, slowly draining your energy reserves—until you find it and fix it.

➢ Check fatigue factor #4 Blood Sugar Imbalance. If your blood sugar is on a roller coaster, this will always impact your cortisol. The two biggest ways you can help smooth out your blood sugar is with diet (Chapter 10) and exercise (Chapter 11).

➢ Because cortisol is related to chronic stress, it is imperative to practice stress management techniques on a daily basis, and add more Vitamin R to your life (Chapter 13).

➢ There is a specific class of herbs known as adaptogens that can help cortisol imbalance. Adaptogenic herbs include:
   ✓ ashwagandha (*Withania somnifera*)

- ✓ Asian ginseng (*Panax ginseng*)
- ✓ Siberian ginseng (*Eleutherococcus senticosus*)
- ✓ rhodiola (*Rhodiola rosea*)
- ✓ holy basil (*Ocimum sanctum*)
➢ Licorice (*Glycyrrhiza glabra*) can be particularly useful to raise cortisol when it's too low (this is why it helps to do a saliva test, so you can see when it is appropriate to use these herbs, especially licorice). But I urge you to use caution with licorice. Taking it too late in the day may keep you up at night. Plus, licorice can raise blood pressure in some people. I recommend whenever you use licorice to monitor your blood pressure on a regular basis.

Chapter 5

Fatigue Factor #4: Blood Sugar Imbalance

Symptoms

When blood sugar is too low, it's called hypoglycemia. When blood sugar is too high, it's called insulin resistance.

Both cause fatigue.

In fact, along with cortisol, blood sugar imbalances are at the top of my functional medicine list as leading causes of fatigue.

If you're not sure if you have low blood sugar, use this questionnaire as your guide.

Hypoglycemia Questionnaire	Yes	No
I crave sweets, especially during the day.		
I get cranky if I miss a meal.		
I depend on coffee to get myself started and/or to keep myself going.		
I get lightheaded if I miss a meal.		
Eating relieves my fatigue.		

I feel shaky if I wait too long to eat.		
I feel agitated, easily upset, nervous between meals.		
I have a poor memory and am forgetful.		

If you have three or more "yes" answers, you are prone to having low blood sugar.

Testing

The HbA1C Test

This blood test is to see if your blood sugar is too high. The HbA1C (hemoglobin A1C) test is also called A1C for short. This test tells you the history of what your blood sugar has been doing over the last three months. The more of a blood sugar roller-coaster ride you're on, the higher your A1C slowly gets. This is hands down a much better test than measuring random or fasting glucose levels, which is what most doctors tend to do.

What's Your A1C?

Ideally your A1C should be at or below 0.054.

If your A1C is 0.055-0.059, your blood sugar is having a hard time keeping in good balance and is most likely contributing to your fatigue. You are also at increased risk of developing pre-diabetes and diabetes in the future if you don't get your A1C at or below 0.054.

If your A1C is 0.060-0.064, you have pre-diabetes. Your blood sugar is definitely not keeping in good balance and *is* contributing to your fatigue. Don't worry! This is very fixable! Your goal is to get your A1C at or below 0.054.

And an A1C at or above 0.065 is diagnostic for diabetes. Your blood sugar is out of control and is a huge part of your fatigue. Don't worry! This is still very fixable! Your goal is to get your A1C at or below 0.054.

Here's a list of the A1C levels for the fatigue patients featured in this book:

A1C Levels Ideal levels are at or below 0.054	
Anne	n/a
Dr. Carri	0.052
Min	0.053
Jocelyne	0.057
Liz	0.059

As you see, two out of four patients had A1C levels above ideal, meaning the blood sugar was starting to become a problem, putting them at increased risk of developing pre-diabetes and diabetes in the future. The above-ideal A1C levels added to their fatigue.

Liz had the worst levels. And, she had been suffering with fatigue for years!

For Liz, food sensitivities—especially a sensitivity to sugar— robbed her energy. Once food became Liz's friend, her energy went from 0 to 100 percent "batteries are on full charge" mode! (Find the cause. Fix the cause. Feel normal again!)

The higher your A1C, the more at risk you are for developing diabetes. A higher A1C will also contribute to hormonal imbalances, high cholesterol, weight gain, chronic pain, and cardiovascular problems. So take this as a lesson in preventative medicine—start now to fix your health or you *will* pay for it later.

Note: A1C is rarely tested by family doctors. Also, as I said previously, whenever you have blood work done, be sure to get a copy of the results for yourself so you can see what your numbers are, what was tested, and what wasn't tested.

Treatment

The fastest and easiest way to control blood sugar imbalances is with diet and exercise. I focus on this in Part 2 of the book.

You May Be Toxic

If you know you already have high blood sugar, pre-diabetes, or even diabetes, and have been working hard on diet and exercise but are seeing little results in your blood work despite all your efforts, you may have too many toxins in your body. (There is a stack of research pointing at environmental toxins as a big underlying cause of insulin resistance, pre-diabetes, and diabetes.) If this is you, it would be wise to find a functional medicine doctor to help you detoxify your body properly and safely.

Oftentimes, it's only after a thorough detoxification program that blood sugar levels finally get back into balance, and you finally get your energy back.

Toxins are not part of my Basic Fatigue List, but are included in my Expanded List. (Again, you can get a free copy of my Expanded List via the Special Bonus section at the end of this book.)

Chapter 6

Fatigue Factor #5: Nutrient Deficiencies

I routinely find at least one of these four nutrients as deficient in my fatigue patients: vitamin B12, vitamin D, magnesium, or iron.

What I find interesting, though, is most women are never checked for all of these nutrients. Sure, your doctor may check one or two of them, but *all* levels should be checked if you want to find the underlying cause of your fatigue.

Remember: Every time you have blood work done, get a copy of the results for yourself. That way you'll know your own numbers and can start tracking them from year to year. Then if a disparity arises, you may catch what a family doctor might overlook.

Vitamin B12 Deficiency

Symptoms

Fatigue is a leading symptom of low B12. Other symptoms can be:

- ➢ weakness
- ➢ lightheadedness
- ➢ pale skin
- ➢ rapid breathing and heartbeat
- ➢ easy bleeding (including gums) or easy bruising

➢ sore tongue
➢ upset stomach
➢ unusual weight loss
➢ diarrhea (or constipation)

Testing

B12 can be measured with a blood test. Ideal levels are above 600 pg/ml. I rarely see this is in my practice, though. Most people do not get enough B12 in their diet, especially if they're not fans of fish and seafood (like me—bring on the grilled steak!).

Here is a list of the B12 levels from the fatigue patients featured in this book:

B12 Levels Ideal is above 600 pg/ml	
Jocelyne	217
Anne	381
Min	396
Liz	441
Dr. Carri	680

As you see, four out of five patients had B12 levels below ideal. Low B12 is quite common.

Jocelyne's B12 was clearly labeled as insufficient on her lab report. One problem—her family doctor never told her about this. No wonder she had fatigue!

Treatment

If you think you're eating enough B12-rich foods, then what it really comes down to is figuring out if the B12 is not getting absorbed properly (like with pernicious anemia or silent Celiac disease), and/or if it's being used up faster than it should be (like with a hidden infection).

Top 10 foods richest in vitamin B12:

1. clams
2. liver
3. kidney
4. beef
5. lamb
6. oysters
7. mackerel
8. crab
9. herring
10. organ meats

B12 is best taken one of two ways: as a painful injection, or as a painless sublingual melt-under-the-tongue lozenge. Studies have compared them head to head, and the results show that the painless sublingual lozenge works just as well as the painful shots.

Besides fatigue, B12 may also be helpful for treating and/or preventing:

- back pain
- muscle cramps
- migraines
- Sciatica
- anxiety
- depression
- poor memory
- diabetes
- infertility
- and much more

Vitamin D Deficiency

Symptoms

Other than fatigue, symptoms of low vitamin D may be vague and somewhat difficult to detect. The symptoms may include:

➢ a general achy feeling in the muscles
➢ moderate pain in the bones

Severe vitamin D deficiency will make those symptoms more pronounced:

➢ muscle weakness
➢ severe pain in the bones
➢ difficulty walking and moving around
➢ dental cavities
➢ increased allergies (in children and adolescents)

Prolonged vitamin D deficiency can contribute or lead to:

➢ severe asthma (in children)
➢ impaired cognitive abilities (in older adults)
➢ stooped posture or deformed bones
➢ cardiovascular disease (can become life threatening)
➢ cancer

Vitamin D deficiency is being talked about as the Grand Deceiver. In an article by Dr. John Cannell, head of the Vitamin D Council, vitamin D deficiency is revealed to mimic or even present as:

➢ sun sensitivity
➢ gingivitis
➢ frequent infections
➢ autoimmune diseases
➢ diabetes

➢ fibromyalgia
➢ stroke
➢ osteoporosis
➢ ankylosing spondylitis (spine-fusing inflammatory disease)

Does any of this sound like you? Or, someone you know? You will never know if you have vitamin D deficiency unless you get tested.

Here is a list of the vitamin D levels from the fatigue patients featured in this book:

Vitamin D Levels Ideally 125-250 nmol/L	
Jocelyne	57
Min	82
Liz	96
Anne	139
Dr. Carri	217

So, three out of five patients had vitamin D levels well below ideal. Like B12, it's very common to have vitamin D deficiency.

Jocelyne's levels were the lowest in our group—a clear deficiency, even by medical standards. Yet Jocelyne's family doctor (who didn't mention her B12 deficiency) never tested her vitamin D!

You can read more about Jocelyne's story next.

Jocelyne's Fatigue Journey—
Listen to Your Gut Feeling; It's Always Right

Dr. Carri: Hello, readers! Today I'm speaking with Jocelyne. Jocelyne, I've known you for many years. You're one of the busiest people I know! And, one of the most successful! I could go on and on about the awards you have won. That's why I was so surprised when you came into my office saying you had terrible fatigue!

Before we get into your story, I want to first thank you for agreeing to share your fatigue journey with our readers. You've always been a helper and a giver—that's part of what makes you so successful in business and in life! I just wanted to take a moment and acknowledge that. Now, are you ready to get started?

Jocelyne: Yes! And you're welcome! And thank you!

Dr. Carri: Tell us about the fatigue that you had. How long did you have it before consulting with me? What other treatments did you try? What other doctors did you see? Generally what was your life like back when you had fatigue?

Jocelyne: Well, I didn't have a life. I literally had to pull myself out of bed in the morning and send the kids to school. Then I would go back to bed and sleep until I had just enough time to get ready for my first appointment. I would always sleep between appointments too. I'd sleep fifteen to sixteen hours per day and was still completely tired.

It all started very slowly, but over the past sixteen months, my energy was just getting worse and worse. In my businesses I just couldn't produce like I used to. I'm very busy—I'm a single mom of two kids, and I also take care of my mother.

I have several businesses. To start with I've been a real estate broker for twenty-five years now. You've seen the awards—I absolutely love my job! But I was barely functioning, and my business was going down and down because I was so tired. My brain was just not there either.

After about a year of this, even the people closest to me started noticing there was something wrong. I was calling them less, seeing them less. I had friends say, "Do you know we haven't seen each other in three months?" That's when I thought, "Okay, there's a problem here!" because I'd rather sleep than be with them!

Even the sports I like—my workout in the morning—I've been doing a workout for years and years. Forty minutes every morning on my treadmill. I could still do it, but I'd go to bed right after! I've been going to Kundalini yoga classes for more than eight years, and I let that go too!

And my kids were noticing my mood. I was less patient, less tolerant. I'm sure my clients also noticed it! Everything was going awry!

I went to see my family doctor for a physical. He didn't find anything wrong.

Two months later I called him back. I said, "Something's wrong with me. This isn't normal." He sent me for a bunch of tests—

blood tests, CT scans, X-rays, MRI…everything. He even sent me to a heart doctor and a neurologist. That's where I got the MRI of the brain, in case I had a tumor in my head.

They couldn't find a thing wrong with me. That's when I knew in my gut, "Go see Carri. She'll know what to do!" So I called your office. I should have done that from the start!

Dr. Carri: Did you have any other symptoms besides the fatigue that you were struggling with? You mentioned your brain. Did you have foggy brain?

Jocelyne: Yes! It was like I was walking inside a cloud. I was really weak too. And weight gain! I gained about twelve pounds.

When you don't have any energy, you also can't think as fast. Usually when people talk to me I'm pretty fast at saying little jokes—that's part of my job. You have to listen at the same time as reading body language and think of what to say next. That's sales, right? I couldn't even do that.

Dr. Carri: Any other symptoms? Bloating? Indigestion?

Jocelyne: Yes, bloating. *Lots* of bloating! I would bloat at least two to three inches through the day, and it hurt! I didn't go to dinner with friends because I knew it would get worse.
Even at home I had to watch everything I was eating. And vacuuming the house—I had to do it in steps because I was getting dizzy. I had *no* energy. I'd never felt like this before!

Dr. Carri: You had fatigue, foggy brain, dizziness, and lots of bloating.

Jocelyne: Yes! And I wasn't sleeping well. I would wake up every night. I'd fall asleep quickly, and then two hours later I'd be awake for three or four hours. How can you function in the day if you can't sleep at night? I'd go back to sleep around five in the morning and have to get up at six with the kids. You can't function like that! It's impossible!

So at night, instead of drinking one glass of wine, I'd drink two to help me sleep. I knew I had to go to bed, and I knew I wouldn't be able to sleep because I had slept most of the day away!

Dr. Carri: Now, you were also waking up at the same time every night too. That's something I want to talk about, because that was a big hint for your fatigue in my opinion.

Jocelyne: It was like clockwork! Between one and one fifteen in the morning, my eyes would open. Months of that!

Dr. Carri: So months of not sleeping well. That's going to have a big domino effect in your body. I told you that waking at the same time every night was a hint for me. It means there is a blockage in your acupuncture channels, particularly the liver channel.

You see, the energy flows through your acupuncture channels, and at different times of the day the energy is concentrated in different areas. It's called the Horary Cycle. At one in the morning, the energy should be shifting from your gallbladder channel to your liver channel. So we added acupuncture to your treatment program to clear the blockage.

Jocelyne, was there anything about having this fatigue that had you really worried, or afraid, or angry?

Jocelyne: Yes, because I couldn't produce. I couldn't be myself!

Dr. Carri: Tell us what you mean by "couldn't produce," because you're a pretty busy real estate broker.

Jocelyne: For me—my whole adult life, I'll say—six or seven hours of sleep is all I've needed.

Dr. Carri: That was normal for you?

Jocelyne: That's normal. I wake up, and I'm completely energized. I do my workout, and then I start my day. Everything goes well. The kids are happy. Time management—I'm pretty good at time management. I would start my dinner in the slow cooker when things were going well. Everybody had good food, everybody was healthy.

Dr. Carri: You're the type of person who cooks everything from scratch too.

Jocelyne: When you work like I do, you have to eat healthy. You can't eat fast food because you'll have a low, and all your hours in a day count—and your brain counts more than anything else, right? If you don't eat right, it's not going to function right. I've never had to control my weight because I've always had an active life.

Dr. Carri: Until all this happened.

Jocelyne: Yes.

Dr. Carri: So you were starting to say that it made you angry because you weren't producing like you used to.

Jocelyne: Yes. And when you see yourself with everything—all the tools and everything—but your body can't follow, it's pretty frustrating. You go to the doctor, and they say you have nothing, or you're depressed, or you're going through a burnout and need a vacation.

Dr. Carri: How did that make you feel?

Jocelyne: I was very mad!

Dr. Carri: When the doctor said you're depressed?

Jocelyne: They couldn't find anything wrong, and he said to me, "You're depressed." I got up—didn't even say good-bye—and I left. I went home, waited a couple of days, and then I called you. I thought, "This is insane! Depressed? I have nothing to be depressed about!"

I know it sounds funny, but I had a gut feeling that it was something I could fix. I knew deep down it was fixable. But how? And where to look? And where to go?

Oh—they also wanted to give me sleeping pills. I don't take any medication. I don't even take aspirin. So, no, I'm not going to take that. Find the *problem* and then we'll see if I want to take the pills. Except they couldn't find the problem!

A total waste of time—that's what I call that year of testing—a waste of time!

When I came to your office, you had my records sent to you, and you saw that my B12 was low! That's when I got really frustrated! It was right there in black and white the whole time, but my doctor never even told me!

Dr. Carri: I have to say that I do find that a lot, and I don't know why; the family doctor will scan through your results, and if there's nothing critically wrong they're just going to ignore it. Whereas for me, these are the exact clues that are needed to solve your case.

Jocelyne: If you're lacking vitamins, your whole body is going to suffer!

Dr. Carri: So for your particular case, your doctor did all of the normal, usual blood work for a patient with fatigue. They'll see if you have an anemia. They'll test your thyroid. They'll check your B12. That's it.

So your doctor did all of the usual things, except your doctor never told you that yes, you actually did have low B12. Low B12 is a very common cause of fatigue.

And then there were some tests that your doctor never ran that we ran. Do you remember that?

Jocelyne: The spitting one?

Dr. Carri: Yes, we did the saliva test for cortisol, and we did some blood work too.

Jocelyne: I'm happy that my gut feeling told me, "This is enough fooling around now. Call Dr. Carri. Call her, and she'll figure it out."

I finally realized I'm so organized with my life, but I didn't take the time or even think of keeping on top of my health. That's very scary, because if you don't have health, you really have nothing. It's the most important one, and we forget about it!

So, you found my B12 was low, and my vitamin D was really low, and my cortisol was out of whack, and I needed acupuncture.

I tell you, it didn't take long before I was sleeping all night. To be honest I was surprised! I'm even telling people to try acupuncture now if they can't sleep!

My kids even said to me, "You look more relaxed. You have more patience." That's where I realized that sleep is a necessity. If you can't sleep, then your whole day and your whole mood and your whole everything is going to be upside down!

Dr. Carri: What was it that made you decide to go ahead with the treatment plan that I suggested? I know you knew me from before and that I'd helped you before....

Jocelyne: It's the questions you asked me. Then you said, "I'm going to have your records sent to me so I can see what was done." After you received my records, you sat down with me and explained what you had found. And then, there was a plan!

There was actually a plan! I've never seen a doctor do that. If there's no plan, how can you fix me?

So, we had a plan. You said to me, "We try this. And if it doesn't work, we modify it." And it worked!

Dr. Carri: How long was it before you noticed improvement? What changed?

Jocelyne: Within two weeks! My vision became better. No more feeling like I was in a cloud. In two weeks it disappeared, so that to me was like, "Whoohooo!" Two weeks was fast!

Dr. Carri: It's not two weeks for everybody. Everybody is different. It's because you never take medication, you already eat a healthy diet, and you exercise daily.

What is life like now that you're better? What do you do now that you couldn't do before?

Jocelyne: I started going out again! I go out with my friends. And for my business, I'm calling clients that last year I was running away from because I didn't have the energy to take on the work. Now my business is growing again. Even some of my clients have said, "You looked so tired before." "Oh, my gosh, you're back!" And the ideas I have! I'm back to my old self! I take my kids skiing every chance I get. We're having fun again. I wasn't fun last year. I was grumpy and I only skied two or three times.

Dr. Carri: What do you see your life like in the future now that you have your energy back?

Jocelyne: Well it can only get better! Or back to what it was, which is still pretty great! I've realized that even though I see my family doctor for a yearly physical, I'm going to ask for the tests and then come see you too, just to maintain my good health.

If you don't take care of yourself, no one else will. And when you're down in the pits—I was lucky because I knew you, but how many people don't? That's why by talking about it, by telling our stories, people will learn through that. We learn from other people's struggles.

I thought fatigue only happened at a certain age, but a week ago I had a client in her thirties, and she's dragging her feet. So I gave her your card and said, "Go and see Dr. Carri. She'll tell you if she can help or not. She'll look at your records. If she can't help you, she'll tell you."

Dr. Carri: Yes, there are a lot of people now with fatigue in their twenties, thirties, forties, and fifties. I even have two patients who are in their seventies. They've always been go-getters with lots of energy throughout their lives, and now their energy is gone. A doctor would say, "You're old. What do you expect?" But they don't buy that excuse. They know there's something wrong, and they want to fix it! I love that attitude!

Do you have any advice for other women struggling with fatigue?

Jocelyne: Yes! To call you! You know fatigue isn't normal. It's not normal to be tired. If it's your diet, if it's your lifestyle—you have to change your lifestyle to have a good life. That results in more energy, being more productive. We all have goals and dreams.

I'm happy. I sleep better. All because of you. So women have to have the energy to do things and to help other people. That's what life is all about. Otherwise, what's the point?

Dr. Carri: Is there anything else that you want to add?

Jocelyne: Unfortunately we're in a healthcare system where every doctor has a job. It doesn't matter how bad they are. They'll still keep their job. And they're all overwhelmed with patients.

Just because you're going through the tests—your blood work, your yearly physical—it doesn't mean that you're actually healthy. If you're tired, you've got to look into it and ask to see your results. Don't let somebody just say "nothing's wrong" when you know there is. You have to listen to yourself. Your gut feeling is always right, except people don't listen to it.

Dr. Carri: So that's the other important point: women need to listen to their gut feelings.

Jocelyne: And that goes back to the basics, right? I'm a believer in natural medicine. I don't take medication. I think doctors are too quick at giving prescriptions. They want to give me prescriptions, but they don't know why they're giving them to me. I even asked my doctor, "Why should I take sleeping pills if you don't even know why I'm waking up at night? I need to know what's causing this."

Dr. Carri: As I say: Find the cause. Fix the cause. Feel normal again! Simple.

Jocelyne: Very easy to say—for you! But for the plain medical doctor it's not. Which means you're not normal! (Laughs.)

Dr. Carri: (Also laughs.) Yes, I'm not normal! I'm a functional medicine doctor! Thank you, Jocelyne, for telling your story!

Jocelyne: You're welcome! But thank you! Because honestly, if it weren't for you, I would not be telling this story with a happy ending!

Think your family doctor has tested you for low vitamin D? Think again.

In Canada, socialized medicine has not covered vitamin D testing for years. And, most family doctors won't test your vitamin D unless you practically beg them to do it. They will say "it's unnecessary; most people are deficient" or "it's an unneeded burden to the healthcare system; laboratories already have enough to do."

Don't believe any of it.

It's your health. Get yourself tested.

At least once a year. Every year.

How do you know if yours has been tested? Ask for a copy of your blood work.

Since vitamin D is not covered by socialized medicine, you have to pay for this test, at least in Canada. So if you haven't shelled out any dollars at the lab, then you haven't been tested.

Testing

Vitamin D can be tested with a blood test. Specifically, 25(OH) vitamin D.

Vitamin D can even be measured from the comfort of your own home. There are labs now that test vitamin D from a simple finger prick and a few drops of blood. (See the Resources section for this information.)

Ideal levels are 125-250 nmol/L (or 50-100 ng/ml; your test will either be in international units or standard units, so look carefully so that you don't get them mixed up!).

Treatment

It's darn near impossible to get vitamin D from your diet alone. Actually, the best source of vitamin D is sunshine. (Here in Ontario where I live, 95 percent of my patients are vitamin D deficient, and 99.9 percent of the doctors here still never check vitamin D levels! Ugh!) So, depending on how much sunshine you get and where you live, you may or may not be making enough vitamin D.

The only way to know is to get your vitamin D checked.

Again, if you want to find the underlying cause of your fatigue, you need to find a doctor trained in functional medicine.

Magnesium Deficiency

Symptoms

Besides fatigue, these are the classic symptoms of magnesium deficiency:

> ➢ crave chocolate

➤ generalized muscle tightness
➤ clench your teeth or grind your teeth at night
➤ twitching in any muscle
➤ muscle cramps or spasms
➤ frequent back pain or back spasms

As you see, many of these classic symptoms have to do with muscles—muscle tightness, muscle twitching, muscle cramps, muscle spasms.

The first time I spoke at the Eastern Ontario Chiropractic Society, I pointed this out. The room was crowded with chiropractors. Of course, one of the biggest complaints patients have about chiropractors is that they have to keep getting adjustments forever, right?

So I explained to them the classic symptoms of magnesium deficiency, and that they would get better and faster results with patients simply by adding magnesium to their treatments.

My other recommendation (and this applies to everyone, not just chiropractors) is always keep a bottle of magnesium on hand in case you throw your back out. It will help get rid of the muscle spasm much faster.

After my presentation, I had twenty minutes of questions, most of them geared toward prescribing magnesium! I was tickled pink that my colleagues were so receptive to the functional medicine approach.

Note: You may also be low in magnesium if you suffer from:

➤ irritability
➤ anxiety
➤ PMS
➤ painful periods

- tension headaches
- migraines
- high blood pressure
- palpitations
- constipation
- fibromyalgia
- restless legs syndrome
- diabetes

Testing

It's estimated that upwards of 80 percent of the population is deficient in magnesium. It's simply no longer in the soil in any abundant amount. Vegetables grown in depleted soil leads to vegetables deficient in nutrients, which leads to a deficiency in your body.

This is one of the few nutrients that I rarely check because it's just cheaper to give my patient a bottle of magnesium to try.

If you prefer a blood test, a serum magnesium test will pretty much always come out normal, unless there is something horribly wrong with your health.

The preferred test for magnesium is called an RBC magnesium. This test measures the amount of magnesium inside the red blood cells.

Best food sources for magnesium:

- raw spinach
- pumpkin seeds
- mackerel
- soybeans
- brown rice
- avocados
- yogurt
- dark chocolate

Treatment

Magnesium comes in different forms. The best form is magnesium glycinate. It's the easiest for your body to absorb, so more ends up in your bloodstream instead of being flushed away.

Iron Deficiency

Symptoms

Besides fatigue, other common symptoms of low iron include:

➤ poor concentration
➤ mood disturbances
➤ cold intolerance
➤ muscle weakness
➤ restless leg syndrome
➤ sore tongue
➤ weak immune system
➤ hair loss

This is a list of the iron (ferritin) levels from the fatigue patients featured in this book:

Ferritin Levels Ideally 40-70 mcg/L	
Min	16
Dr. Carri	23
Liz	47
Anne	48
Jocelyne	75

Two out of five patients had iron levels significantly below ideal.

Min had the worst levels. Yet, despite her chronic fatigue, her doctor kept telling her all her blood tests were normal.

Testing

Family doctors frequently test for ferritin, but not always.

Iron is measured with a ferritin blood test. As noted in the Ferritin Levels chart, ideal levels of ferritin are 40-70 mcg/L. Iron is interesting in that it can be too low or too high. Both can cause fatigue.

Iron that is too low doesn't always get found with an anemia test (a CBC test), so a good doctor will check your ferritin separately.

How do you know if yours has been tested? Ask for a copy of your blood work. You will see if you've been tested, and what your numbers are.

Treatment

When iron is too low, you need to find the reason *why* and not just start supplementing with iron. The most common reasons for low iron that medical doctors don't routinely check for are H. pylori infection in the stomach, silent Celiac disease, small intestinal bacterial overgrowth (SIBO), and parasitic infection.

Please note: Do *not* take iron supplements unless you know what your ferritin level is first. This is one of the few supplements that will build up in your body and damage it beyond repair.

IF YOU HAVE CHRONIC IRON DEFICIENCY...

If you have been suffering with low iron for years or if low iron runs in your family, consider you may actually have Celiac disease or a gluten sensitivity (see text box) preventing the absorption of iron. Low iron is commonly the very first sign of Celiac disease and gluten sensitivity.

And, for those of you who have tried and tried to get your iron levels up with supplements but it just isn't working, you most likely have SIBO (small intestinal bacteria overgrowth)—bacteria are eating the iron and stealing it from you. (This can be diagnosed with a breath test.)

> If you suffer with fatigue and foggy brain, you may have undiagnosed gluten sensitivity.
>
> Gluten sensitivity is not part of my Basic Fatigue List, but it is included in my Expanded List. You can get a free copy of my Expanded List via the Special Bonus section at the end of this book.

You can read more about SIBO in Chapter 7: Chronic Infections.

Note: With both of the above scenarios (Celiac disease and SIBO), it's important to make sure your family doctor has ruled out all other causes of iron deficiency, like a bleeding ulcer, or a bleeding polyp, or even cancer.

IS YOUR FATIGUE FROM TOO MUCH IRON?

Fatigue is most often associated with low iron levels. But not always. Your fatigue may be from too much iron.

Iron that's too high is called iron overload, or hemochromatosis.

> ➢ Ferritin >199 mcg/L in women is suggestive of iron overload.
> ➢ Ferritin >299 mcg/L in women and men is most likely iron overload.
> ➢ Ferritin >799 mcg/L is practically diagnostic of iron overload.

Elevated ferritin should always be confirmed by retesting, and then investigated further as to the underlying cause (which is often silent inflammation or silent infections, but can also be genetic). Find the cause. Fix the cause. Feel normal again!

Iron that is too high will get stored in your heart, liver, pancreas, and in your joints, slowly damaging the tissues beyond repair. Once it's there, it's hard to get out. You don't want this when it's completely treatable.

Please note once again: Do *not* take iron supplements unless you know what your ferritin level is first. This is one of the few supplements that will build up in your body and damage it beyond repair.

How Do I Know If My Supplements Are Working? Try the Vinegar Test!

Most new patients who come to see me are already taking vitamin supplements. In fact, they're usually taking the right supplements! The problem is they either are not taking a strong enough dose in order to have a therapeutic effect, or their supplements are not dissolving and end up in the toilet instead of their bloodstream.

You've probably heard the stories about vitamin supplements. Whole tablets being seen in the intestines on x-rays. Whole tablets being found routinely in septic systems.

How do you know if your vitamin tablets are dissolving or just ending up down the plumbing pipes? Aside from examining your stool (which you could do, but I bet you won't!) there's an easier test you can do.

The vinegar test.

This is how it works. The acid in your stomach is a pH of 1.5 to 3.5. The acid content of white vinegar is a pH of about 2.4. This means you can use plain old white vinegar to see if your vitamin tablets dissolve or not.

If they dissolve in the white vinegar, they will most likely dissolve in your stomach too. (Unless you use acid blocking medications, in which case this entire experiment doesn't hold true. See the next section, Are Acid Blockers Robbing You of Nutrients?, to learn more.)

So, to a clear glass, add ¼ cup white vinegar, then a vitamin tablet. Set your timer for thirty minutes.

If at the end of thirty minutes:

a. the tablet has not dissolved, it will probably not dissolve in your stomach either, and will end up straight in your toilet. That tablet is garbage and a waste of money. Find a better supplement.

b. the tablet has dissolved completely, it should dissolve completely in your stomach too.

c. the tablet has only partially dissolved, poke at it with your finger and see if it will break down more. (In reality, the movement of your stomach churning your food will help break the tablet down.) But if the tablet is still rock hard, the rest of it will probably end up languishing in the sewer. In that case, it's garbage and you need to find a better supplement.

Until I heard about the vinegar test, I relied on the kindness of my vitamin reps who always told me, "All our supplements are pharmaceutical grade and are rigorously tested for dissolvability and absorption," or "We only use the highest standards for making sure our tablets dissolve."

Then I did the vinegar test on all the supplements I took that were in tablet form. And I was shocked at what I found.

Some of the tablets dissolved completely. These I kept in my vitamin dispensary.

Many of the tablets dissolved partially but at the core were still rock hard. Some of the tables didn't dissolve *at all*. (And these tablets were from some of the most expensive supplement companies too!) I got rid of all these.

The vinegar test works best on tablets. Sure, you could test your capsules, but save your time—capsules always dissolve.

That should give you a hint: Supplements work best in capsule (or powder or liquid) forms. They are the easiest for your body to break down and absorb, compared to tablets. More ends up in your bloodstream instead of down your toilet!

In my dispensary, 99 percent of the supplements I now carry are capsules.

Are Acid Blockers Robbing You of Nutrients? Beware of PPIs!

Acid blocking medications, specifically proton pump inhibitors, or PPIs, are well-known causes of nutrient deficiencies.

What does a PPI do? It blocks the acid in your stomach.

In order to absorb the nutrients from your food and your supplements, you need to have a strong acid environment in your stomach. Without strong stomach acid, most nutrients end up—well, you know—instead of in your bloodstream.

What a waste.

These are all proton pump inhibitors:

> ➢ omeprazole (Prilosec)

- ➤ rapid release omeprazole (Zegerid)
- ➤ esomeprazole (Nexium)
- ➤ lansoprazole (Prevacid)
- ➤ dexlansoprazole (Dexilant)
- ➤ rabeprazole (Aciphex)
- ➤ pantoprazole (Protonix)

Are you taking any of these medications? If so, has your doctor warned you about the dangers of PPIs?

Long-term use of PPIs increases your risk of developing:

- ➤ food allergies
- ➤ infections of the digestive tract
- ➤ stomach cancer
- ➤ colon cancer
- ➤ osteopenia
- ➤ osteoporosis
- ➤ fractures of the hip, spine, forearm, and wrist
- ➤ pneumonia
- ➤ acute kidney failure

Note: "Long-term use" can be as little as *90 days* on a PPI!

PPI Research (a partial list)

- ➤ According to a Danish study, the occurrence of stomach cancer is directly related to the amount of PPI prescription refills and the length of use (Poulsen AH et al, 2009).
- ➤ Women over age fifty who take PPIs for more than a year have a 44 percent increased risk of hip fracture (Geller JL, 2007).
- ➤ Long-term PPI therapy, particularly at high doses, is associated with an increased risk of hip fracture by 245 percent (Geller JL, 2007).

➢ Women's Health Initiative study showed a modest association between PPI use and increased risk of spine, forearm, and wrist fracture (Gray SL et al, 2010).

➢ In 2010 the FDA revised the labeling of all PPIs to include the increased risk of fractures of the hip, wrist, and spine.

➢ NSAIDs (nonsteroidal anti-inflammatory drugs) are the number one cause of acute kidney failure. PPIs are the number two cause (Raza MN et al, 2012).

PPIs and Nutrient Deficiencies

Without proper stomach acid levels, the ability to properly digest and absorb nutrients is significantly impaired. Specifically:

➢ Calcium deficiency—With a PPI, proper digestion of calcium plummets from 96 percent down to 23 percent (O'Connell et al 2005).

➢ B12 deficiency—PPI use (past and present) is significantly associated with the presence of B12 deficiency (Lam JR et al 2013).

➢ Magnesium deficiency—All PPIs are associated with magnesium depletion. Esomeprazole (Nexium) had the lowest risk, and pantoprazole (Protonix) had the highest risk. The risk is higher in males and the elderly. Low calcium and low potassium are also commonly found, along with low magnesium, as a side effect of PPIs (Luk CP et al, 2013).

➢ Iron deficiency—Iron malabsorption is especially affected in patients who are iron deficient before starting on a PPI (Sharma VR, 2004).

Rebound Acidity

PPIs cause significant rebound acidity. This can happen within as little as three months after starting on a PPI. This is why most people feel like they can never stop their PPIs. As soon as they miss a dose or two, their stomach acidity increases dramatically and they feel significant burning, indigestion, and reflux, so they swallow down another PPI pill to stop the burn. And the cycle continues.

In fact, research shows that this rebound acid hypersecretion lasts from eight to twenty-six weeks after long-term PPI use is stopped ("long-term use" being three months or more).

How to Safely Get Off Your PPI

To safely get off your PPI, follow these steps one by one.

1. Ask your prescribing doctor about discontinuing your PPI.
2. Find a functional medicine doctor to help you. He or she will help strengthen your stomach lining, reduce inflammation, and get your stomach to function normally again with proper diet, herbs, and nutrients (find the cause, fix the cause, so you stomach works normally again!) while your prescribing doctor slowly weans you off your PPI.
3. Ask your prescribing doctor for the lowest PPI dose available.
4. Ask your prescribing doctor if you can decrease your dose to an every-other-day dosage.
5. Ask your prescribing doctor if you can then go to an every-third-day dosage.
6. Ask your prescribing doctor to switch you to an H2 blocker if you are still having symptoms with acidity.

Remember: Rebound hyperacidity can last from eight weeks to twenty-six weeks after discontinuing PPI use, so time and patience is required to get through this process.

Get your free copy of "Six Truths You Need to Hear about Natural Treatments for Fatigue...Like It or Not" at www.FeelNormalAgainBook.com/SpecialBonus

Chapter 7

Fatigue Factor #6: Chronic Infections

A chronic infection can and will drain your body of nutrients and energy.

By chronic infection I mean a chronic, silent, hidden, underlying infection deep in your body. This can be from too much bad bacteria, a parasite infestation, yeast overgrowth, or not enough good bacteria (probiotics).

Hidden infections are very common. Have you ever had food poisoning? Have you ever had a twenty-four-hour flu or a stomach flu? Have you traveled outside of the country and gotten sick? Answering yes to one of these questions may be a clue to solving your fatigue.

Symptoms

Antibiotics are a leading cause of chronic infections.

Think about this: Usually when women take antibiotics, they end up with a vaginal yeast infection, right? This is because the antibiotics killed off the bad bacteria *and* a whole bunch of the good bacteria too.

If you have a vaginal yeast infection, you're lucky—in the sense that you've found the yeast infection. But what if that yeast infection ends up in your intestines instead of your vagina? You won't feel it, and it will be there for years draining your energy. This is what I mean by a hidden chronic infection caused by antibiotics.

So, how many times in your life have you been on antibiotics? Is there a history of antibiotic use six to twelve months prior to your fatigue starting? If yes, then you may have found the underlying cause of your fatigue.

Antibiotics can cause chaos in the intestines for up to four years!

That's *one* round of antibiotics! How many rounds have you been on in your life?

Many women have chronic infections, and this contributes to their fatigue. The problem is the infection very, very rarely shows up on any blood work. And when there are signs of an infection on the blood work, it usually gets ignored by the doctor unless you're having fever, diarrhea, and vomiting.

My patient Maria is proof of this. She had been on multiple rounds of antibiotics throughout her adult life, for ear infections and bladder infections. She also had multiple yeast infections. When she came to see me, she was suffering with chronic pain all over and terrible fatigue.

Testing

Like I do with all patients, I requested Maria's recent blood work from her family doctor. What I saw shocked me. For at least three years, her white blood cells were low, and steadily declining. Maria's doctor never told her about this. He always said, "Everything's normal."

Now, your white blood cells are like soldiers—they attack invaders to your body, like infections. The problem with Maria was that her soldiers were losing the war and the infections were winning.

I was so concerned with Maria's terrible blood work that I sent her back to her family doctor for a full work up. Frankly, I was afraid she had cancer or something worse. But after multiple trips to her family doctor, and even a rheumatologist, she was still told "everything's normal."

I knew we had to hunt down Maria's infection. I did stool testing and found *four* infections—two bacteria, a yeast, and a fungus—all slowly decimating Maria's white blood cells.

Once the infections were cleared from her body, her white blood cells went back to normal, and Maria finally started to feel better.

Stool Testing

The easiest and best test to evaluate for hidden infections in the colon is a stool test. Not all stool tests are the same, though. You want a test that requires three to four stool samples. This is because parasites, in particular, live in cycles. They are not always found in each and every bowel movement. Also, parasites cling to the walls of the intestines and rarely get shed into the stool. This is another reason why multiple stool samples need to be collected for best test results.

Stool testing is one of the most expensive tests to do, but the investment is worth it. It very often uncovers the underlying reason why you have fatigue.

Hint: If you're doing a stool test, take a laxative formula that will induce watery diarrhea (like for a colonoscopy test). Collect your stool starting after the fourth watery bowel movement. This will increase your chances of finding parasites. If your test calls for 4 samples, consider doubling it by filling each vial halfway twice, thereby collecting 8 samples total in your 4 vials.

Breath Testing

Stool testing tests what's living in the colon, but what about what's living in the small intestine?

Actually, there should be very, very little bacteria living in your small intestine. It should all be in your colon.

However, a common cause of fatigue is bacterial overgrowth in the small intestine, called SIBO (small intestinal bacterial overgrowth). The easiest and best test to evaluate for SIBO is a breath test—the Lactulose Breath Test.

Lactulose is a carbohydrate that doesn't get absorbed by your body. Lactulose is actually food for the bacteria living inside your intestines. So when you take lactulose, the bacteria in your intestines eat it and convert it into gas—hydrogen or methane gas primarily.

Then you breathe out these gases so they can be measured. Depending on how fast the gases are formed, we will know if they are from bacteria in the small intestine or colon.

SIBO is extremely common, especially for those who have fatigue as well as IBS (irritable bowel syndrome)!

Ever Wondered if You Really Have IBS or Not?

Properly diagnosing IBS can be difficult. It relies on a questionnaire along with ruling out other intestinal diseases, like colitis and Celiac disease.

Following is the questionnaire, called the Rome III questionnaire.

(Take a moment to answer it yourself, and then have all your family members take the test.)

Rome III Questionnaire

Have you had <u>recurrent abdominal pain or discomfort</u> at least 3 days per month in the last 3 months associated with <u>2 or more</u> of the following:

1. improvement with defecation
2. onset associated with a change in frequency of stool
3. onset associated with a change in appearance of stool

If your answer is "yes," then you most likely have IBS and SIBO.

SIBO also commonly causes:

> ➢ rosacea
> ➢ fatty liver
> ➢ restless leg syndrome
> ➢ fibromyalgia
> ➢ chronic pain (especially if you've used painkillers and anti-inflammatory medications longer than three months)

If any of this sounds like you, consider getting tested for SIBO. This may be the underlying cause for your fatigue!

Treatment

With chronic infections, curative treatments will vary. Many medical doctors will want to prescribe even more medications, which is often what *caused* the chronic infection in the first place. Be sure to consult with a functional medicine doctor!

Chapter 8

Fatigue Factor #7: Hidden Food Allergies & Sensitivities

Hidden food allergies and sensitivities are known as the "great mimickers." A food allergy or sensitivity can trigger any symptom in your body, including your fatigue!

It's highly likely that you have at least one hidden food allergy or sensitivity, if not *many* more. I'm going to help you find them.

First, let me explain the differences between allergies and sensitivities, because there's a lot of confusion and misinformation on the subject.

Allergies versus Sensitivities

Allergies and sensitivities all have to do with reactions from the immune system.

Think of your immune system like the military. There are different branches of the military, and they each serve a unique and specific purpose—Army, Navy, Air Force, Marines, and Special Forces.

Just as there are different branches of the military, there are also different branches of the immune system. When it comes to allergies and sensitivities, they are known as IgE, IgA, and IgG reactions.

(There are also IgD and IgM, but since they cannot be tested yet, I will leave them out of the discussion for now.)

IgE reactions are food allergies. IgA and IgG reactions are food sensitivities.

Food Allergies

Without getting overly technical, a food allergy is an IgE response from the immune system. In fact, the term *allergy* is medically defined as an IgE reaction.

This is the branch of the immune system that only allergists will deal with.

Symptoms

An IgE reaction to a food is considered a true allergy and is the strongest of all the immune reactions. An example of this is when a person eats strawberries and then immediately breaks out in hives. Or, when a person eats peanuts and develops a life threatening allergic response.

But not all IgE food allergies will show this immediate amount of strength. A person can have multiple IgE food allergies without even knowing it! And this may be an underlying cause of your fatigue.

Testing

A suspected food allergy is usually tested with a skin prick test by an allergist.

Unfortunately, the skin prick test only finds about 50 percent of IgE food allergies. So if you have already seen an allergist and had a skin prick test done, that's a good start. But you're not done yet.

The next step would be to get an IgE blood test done for food allergies. Panels are commonly done for 95, 150, even 300 plus foods.

Now that you understand what a food allergy is (an IgE response), let's briefly look at IgA and IgG.

Food Sensitivities

Symptoms

The next level down in response is the IgA and IgG reactions—food sensitivities.

In addition to fatigue, food sensitivities can cause:

> ➤ runny nose
> ➤ digestive upsets
> ➤ skin rashes
> ➤ headaches
> ➤ depression
> ➤ anxiety
> ➤ foggy brain
> ➤ constipation
> ➤ diarrhea

The reaction you're looking for can be one or more of the above, or anything unusual for you. It can be as simple as a racing heartbeat. Any reaction to a food means you have a problem with that food.

Testing

Food sensitivities can be tested with blood, but sensitivities are tricky to find. They tend to wax and wane, depending on how much of the food you have eaten during the weeks before the test is run.

They also wax and wane depending on how much irritation is already going on deep inside your intestines. The more irritation in your intestines, the more sensitivities tend to show up on a test.

On top of that—and here is a little secret that most doctors aren't even aware of—most labs will use foods in their *raw* form to test with.

This is fine for fruits and veggies. But, testing to see if you are allergic to raw pork? Or raw shellfish? Or raw oats? You would never eat that stuff raw!

When we cook our foods, it changes their chemical structure, which would also mean it would generate an immune response altogether different from raw foods. See the problem?

Here's another gem. You may be fine with (not sensitive to) individual foods, but start combining them together and you may get a whole different scenario. Take pizza for example. You may show no sensitivities to tomato, mozzarella, wheat, yeast, or oregano, but combine them all together and now you have a different beast that you may be sensitive to. Obviously it would be impossible to test for combinations of foods.

Unfortunately there is no best way to test for IgG and IgA food sensitivities via blood work. There will always be some false positives (showing a sensitivity when you really have none), and there will always be false negatives (doesn't show a reaction even though you do actually have a sensitivity).

Having said all of that (hang in there!)...

Yes, the technology for testing IgG and IgA food sensitivities is not 100 percent. But, it is the best we have right now. So as long as you understand the pros and cons of the test first, you can at least make an informed decision about having yourself tested or not.

Lastly, IgA and IgG reactions are never tested by allergists. Allergists only deal with IgE skin prick tests. Functional medicine doctors are the ones who will test all three—IgE, IgA, and IgG.

(Phew—thanks for hanging in there!)

Now, let's get back to resolving your fatigue!

Treatment for Food Allergies and Sensitivities

The Most Common Food Sensitivities

You can be sensitive to nearly anything. However, the most common food sensitivities are (in order):

- ➢ wheat
- ➢ orange
- ➢ eggs
- ➢ tea
- ➢ coffee
- ➢ chocolate

➢ milk
➢ beef
➢ corn
➢ cane sugar
➢ yeast

To find what you're sensitive to:

Option 1: Avoid everything on this list and see if that helps your fatigue.

OR

Option 2: You may want to get the blood testing done for IgE, IgA, and IgG food reactions. It's definitely the most expensive option. But if you're like me and don't want to tinker with your diet unless you really have to, then have the blood test done. You'll have your answers in two to three weeks.

OR

Option 3: Actually the best way to detect food allergies and sensitivities is to do an Elimination Diet, followed by a Food Challenge.

The Elimination Diet

The Elimination Diet/Food Challenge goes like this. Eliminate all those foods listed above (and more, if you like), and eat a very clean diet for two to three weeks. Then, slowly reintroduce the foods you have been avoiding, one at a time, to see if you have a reaction to anything.

You need to wait seventy-two hours in between each new food introduction, because food reactions can be delayed up to seventy-two hours. (This is precisely the reason you can be sensitive to something you eat every day but not even realize it!)

Although the Elimination Diet is considered the best way to assess for hidden food sensitivities, it's time consuming and requires a certain attention to detail that many people just cannot add into their already busy lives.

Liz's story is a perfect example of how hidden food sensitivities can cause your fatigue (you'll find her story ahead in Chapter 10). She had fatigue, foggy brain, chronic pain, and insomnia. Liz did a basic Elimination Diet and found fourteen food sensitivities. Fourteen!

Find the cause. Fix the cause. Feel normal again!

Chapter 9

Fatigue Factor #8: Brain Chemical Imbalance

Your fatigue could literally be all in your head.

By this I mean your brain chemistry might be out of balance, causing your fatigue. This was the case with Anne's fatigue and my fatigue.

There are many different brain chemicals, or neurotransmitters, but for our purposes I'll talk about two: serotonin and dopamine.

Serotonin

Serotonin you've probably already heard of. It's the "feel good, keep you happy and content" neurotransmitter. It primarily regulates mood, appetite, and sleep.

Serotonin is made from the building block 5-HTP, which is an amino acid.

Symptoms

When serotonin levels are low, common symptoms are (in addition to fatigue):

> ➤ poor memory and concentration
> ➤ sugar cravings

➢ weight gain and difficulty losing weight
➢ unstable moods
➢ sadness
➢ depression
➢ anxiety
➢ worrying
➢ poor sleep

Serotonin imbalance can also cause:

➢ migraines
➢ irritable bowel syndrome
➢ ulcerative colitis
➢ Crohn's disease
➢ sex hormone imbalances

Dopamine

Dopamine is the other main neurotransmitter. Dopamine helps keep you mentally focused, with good concentration and good memory. Dopamine in made from the amino acid tyrosine.

Symptoms

When dopamine levels are low, common symptoms are similar to low serotonin. In addition to fatigue you might feel:

➢ lack of mental focus/poor concentration
➢ cravings or intense cravings
➢ weight gain and difficulty losing weight
➢ depression
➢ tremors
➢ restless legs
➢ low self-confidence

Dopamine imbalance can also cause:

➢ addictive behaviors
➢ compulsive tendencies (OCD)
➢ restless leg syndrome
➢ tremors
➢ Parkinson's symptoms

Testing Serotonin and Dopamine

Brain Balancing—MTO Testing

Brain Balancing—MTO testing offers great promise for treating fatigue from a natural medicine standpoint.

MTO stands for monoamine transporter optimization. It's a mouthful, I know. Monoamines are serotonin and dopamine…your brain chemicals.

Without getting too technical, this is basically a way to assess your dopamine and serotonin levels with simple urine testing. You take a prescribed amount of amino acid supplements for a week, and then collect your urine for testing.

Treatment for Serotonin and Dopamine

Brain Balancing—MTO

Depending on how your body reacted to the amino acid supplements, a new recipe of amino acids may be prescribed for a week, and then another urine test is run.

Testing and treatment continue in this manner until the "brain balancing formula" for you is found.

By "brain balancing formula," I mean the right cocktail of balanced amino acids to keep your serotonin and dopamine at optimal levels. This cocktail varies from person to person, and actually does not depend on the severity of the fatigue.

(You can learn about my experience with the Brain Balancing Program and my fatigue story just ahead.)

If you have any of the symptoms of serotonin or dopamine deficiency besides fatigue, even if it's just a foggy brain, then Brain Balancing—MTO testing may be the cure for your fatigue.

Eat Protein

Part of treating brain chemical imbalances is to make sure you're eating enough protein in your diet, since protein is the source of the amino acids that make your neurotransmitters. If you aren't eating enough protein, you won't have adequate construction materials to make your brain chemicals.

This gets particularly important for those who are vegetarian or vegan, and for those who have a hard time digesting protein. But it really applies to everyone.

How much protein you should be eating depends on your level of activity. The more active you are, the more protein you will need.

To calculate how much protein you require, take your ideal body weight (in pounds), and multiply that by the number that corresponds to your activity level:

Recommended Grams of Protein Per Pound of Body Weight Per Day	
Sedentary adult	0.4
Adult recreational exerciser	0.5-0.75
Adult competitive athlete	0.6-0.9
Adult building muscle mass	0.7-0.9
Dieting athlete	0.7-1.0

Example: Mary weighs 150 pounds and is sedentary. Her daily protein requirement would be:

150 x 0.4 = 60 grams of protein daily.

I recommend you calculate your personal protein requirements. Then, roughly calculate your protein consumption for a week, and see if you're getting the protein you require. You can easily do an Internet search for a food protein content chart to find many good sources of protein.

If you're not digesting protein well (you may notice gas, bloating, or indigestion after high-protein meals; a full feeling after eating only a little; or the sensation of food stuck and not moving in your gut), you may consider adding a digestive enzyme supplement with your meals.

Congratulations for reading this far! That truly is a lot to "absorb" (I just had to throw that in). You now know the eight most common causes of fatigue and their treatments, and are on your way to finally feeling normal energy again!

Find the cause. Fix the cause. Feel normal again!

The crowd goes wild!

And the best is yet to come. Up next, immediately following my fatigue story, are tips (some you might not have even heard of before!) to help you build a foundation for *lasting* energy.

My Fatigue Journey— I Didn't Think It Would Ever Happen to ME!

Fatigue is one of the most common complaints in my office. I would say that four out of five new patients have fatigue in their top three complaints.

I just didn't think it would ever happen to me!

My fatigue started in 2009. I was celebrating fifteen years in practice as a chiropractor, but I wasn't happy in my career. It wasn't as fulfilling as I had always hoped. So in 2009 I decided to go back to school—naturopathic school.

It was a tough decision. I moved from Canada to Chicago, leaving my husband, my dogs, and my patients behind. They all gave me their full support, and I needed it!

In Chicago I asked for the biggest course load they could give me in order to get back to Canada in less than two years. Since I was already a doctor, they allowed this.

I loaded my schedule full of courses. I was in class thirty hours a week—morning, afternoon, *and* evening classes. Add to that study time, writing term papers, giving presentations, and preparing for exams (there were a lot of those!).

On top of that, I was traveling back and forth to Canada at least once a month to treat my patients. I took classes all week, and then Friday afternoon I would leave for the airport. I'd arrive in Ottawa Friday night, work all day Saturday from nine to five and Sunday from eight to noon seeing patients, then it was straight back to the airport and back in Chicago Sunday night so I didn't miss class Monday morning.

It was an insane schedule! And a lot of pressure to succeed. Thinking back on it, I don't even know how I did it all! I was the definition of "burning the candle at both ends."

This was one of the most stressful times of my life. Lots of late nights, lots of tossing and turning, lots of knots in my stomach, lots of coffee to make it through my day. I'll also say it was one of the best decisions that I made in my life too. But definitely it was stressful!

About six months in was when the fatigue really hit me.

In the beginning I just shrugged it off because I knew the fatigue was because of stress. At one point I came back to Canada between semesters and went to my family doctor for my yearly checkup. She ran the usual blood work. Then I got a call to come back in and see her, so I knew something was wrong in my blood work.

She said my thyroid was low and followed that up with, "We'll just watch it. I'm sure it's nothing."

I said, "Whoa, whoa, whoa—wait a second. What do you mean my thyroid is low? How low is low?"

My TSH was 7.15. Ideal is under 2.0, so I knew this was bad.

The next thing she said was, "We don't usually do anything about this until your numbers are into the double digits."

And I thought, "*What?* That makes no sense! You're just going to wait until I get worse before you'll do something about it?"

I asked for more testing—to find the cause. Actually, it was more like a debate, because that concept—find the cause—seemed foreign to my doctor. (I honestly don't mean to doctor bash. They do their best, but their hands are tied by the system. So it can be really frustrating, even for me, to deal with doctors.)

From a functional medicine standpoint, the two most common reasons for low thyroid are 1) high cortisol levels due to stress (the most likely scenario for me), and 2) the autoimmune thyroid condition Hashimoto's Thyroiditis (also a possibility for me since I'm a woman in the prime years for autoimmune disease to pop up).

I said, "Okay, I want to find the cause of this. I want to do some testing to rule out Hashimoto's. I want to do antibody testing—thyroperoxidase antibodies and thyroglobulin antibodies—and a vitamin D test."

She said, "No. It's not necessary."

I dug my heels in further. And then I spewed out the physiology of the immune system, the biochemistry of the thyroid hormones, and the actions of vitamin D, and why these are all so important if I had Hashimoto's. Then I explained again why I wanted these extra tests run.

Honestly, I think she just gave in to shut me up!

The test showed I didn't have Hashimoto's, so that left me in the cortisol and stress scenario as the cause of my low thyroid.

I thought, "All right. I'll take better care of myself." I started a vitamin and herb regimen. Then I headed back to the grind of school.

All the stress, stress, stress just kept accumulating. In my head I told myself, "Carri, this is just short-term pain for long-term gain. You just have to suck it up! Suck it up so that you can get that diploma and practice natural medicine. This is your dream. Just keep your eye on the prize!"

So that's what I did.

I worked extra hard, paid my dues, and slowly counted down the days until graduation!

By the time that day came, my batteries were nearly dead. After graduation I basically slept for three months. I would sleep ten hours at night and take a two-hour nap every afternoon. I thought, "This is what I need to recharge my batteries. I just need to sleep because I've put my body through too much stress. Sleep will fix it."

Then came board exams. More studying. More stress. More sleepless nights. And more pressure than ever! "I have to pass my boards. I have to pass my boards." In the end, I graduated valedictorian of my class. I had put *so* much pressure on myself!

After my board exams, I was back to sleeping ten hours per night and two-hour naps every afternoon. Except this didn't recharge my batteries. At all.

Months went by, and my fatigue still wasn't any better. I started taking more supplements, more herbs, more everything. It helped, but only a little.

Once my ND license arrived, I could start testing myself. I could really apply functional medicine to myself. The first thing I did was a saliva test for cortisol. These are my cortisol results:

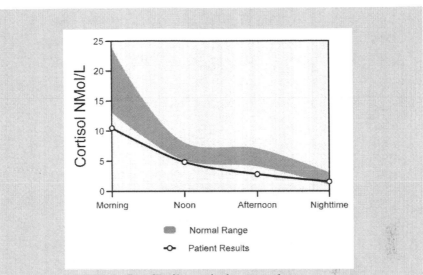

Dr. Carri's cortisol test results

My cortisol was low all day long. I was in Stage 3 Adrenal Exhaustion. No wonder I had so much fatigue! This definitely changed my treatment approach with the vitamins and herbs I was taking. I also started a gluten-free diet.

After seven or eight weeks, my energy was a little better, but I still had a long way to go. So the next thing I did was a stool test. Bingo! I found a parasite! Cryptosporidium parvum, a very common parasite. I probably got it from my dogs. They lick everything, including me. I treated the parasite with herbs.

My energy got a little better again, and my psoriasis totally cleared up (I had been battling that for more than ten years!), but I knew I still had a ways to go.

Besides the fatigue, I was also struggling with my brain. I think going back to school fried my brain! Seriously! Stress—or cortisol—actually does kill off brain cells. I had foggy brain, poor memory, lack of concentration, lack of motivation, lack of drive, and I was distracted easily. I had to rely on sticky notes and lists, otherwise I would forget. I would ask my husband a question and forget his answer, so I'd ask the question again. He would get upset and thought I wasn't listening to him.

The reality was my brain just wasn't working! I felt like I had adult ADD—attention deficit disorder. I'd start one little project, and I'd get distracted and go to something else, and then I'd get distracted again and go on to another thing. And nothing was actually getting done!

I was worried. As a doctor I really rely on my critical thinking skills, especially with functional medicine. I was also getting angry. Why did I still have fatigue? Why couldn't I fix myself? Would I ever be normal again?

The last piece of my fatigue puzzle was fixing my brain. I signed up to learn the Brain Balancing Program by Dr. Dan Kalish. (Actually he calls it the Mind Mapping Program, but I like Brain Balancing Program better, so that's what I call it.)

I treated myself first. Who better to be the guinea pig, right? With the Brain Balancing Program, you take a series of amino acid supplements and do urine tests until you determine the right combination of amino acids that keeps your serotonin and dopamine at optimal levels. It's a lot of capsules to swallow, and the testing can be rigorous. But once I found the right combination for me, it was like a light bulb turned on inside my brain! All the neurons were firing again, the world seemed brighter, my brain was clear, and I felt fully present again. I felt like my old self!

It was the most amazing feeling! It's really hard to describe in words, but I felt like, "Okay! I'm back at 100 percent! My brain is back online!" My fatigue was finally gone. I finally felt normal again.

Being on those amino acid supplements to keep my brain in balance—that was the biggest part of my fatigue puzzle.

So what's my life like now that my fatigue is gone? Well, I get a lot more done. Like this book, for one! And I'm more focused at the office and in my business. I'm exercising every day, which I didn't do for a long time. I'm out there walking my Basset hounds. I just enjoy life more. And I don't sleep my life away anymore either.

I've always had lots of plans and goals and dreams that I've wanted to achieve. Now I can see they are achievable again.

My advice for other women struggling with fatigue is don't give up! You should always have hope. There *is* a reason why you have fatigue.

My other advice is be patient. Fatigue takes time to figure out.

For most patients there are multiple reasons why the fatigue is there. Like for me—the low cortisol, the gluten sensitivity, the parasite infection, the brain imbalance. That took a lot of time to figure out, let alone fix.

Sometimes it really can be a needle in a haystack. But that needle is there, waiting to be found, and when you keep digging for it, you *will* eventually find it! And then feel normal again, and get your health back, and get your life back!

You've got to find the cause, and then fix the cause, so that you can feel normal again. Find a functional medicine doctor to work with. They will help find the needle in your fatigue haystack.

Thank you for reading my story. I hope it helps you or someone you love

Dr. Cain

Part 2

Build Your Foundation for *Lasting* Energy

Chapter 10

Energize Your Lifestyle

With all the information you gleaned in the first part of the book, you're now on the road to discovering the originating cause of your fatigue, fixing the cause, and feeling normal again.

But, did you know that what you do every day probably makes your fatigue worse?

What you eat and drink has a huge impact on your energy levels. So does stress, sleep, exercise, and something I like to call vitamin R—rest, relaxation, and recreation.

There are many things that are not in your control, but your lifestyle isn't one of them. Simple lifestyle changes may be your ticket to lasting energy. I've had some of the toughest cases of fatigue turn right around by applying the lifestyle changes that I list in the pages ahead. It's true!

You can spend buckets of money on testing and buckets more on supplements, but if your lifestyle is crap, you will only get so far with your fatigue.

In functional medicine we want to do testing to find the cause of your fatigue, but then we need to make sure we build a strong foundation for health. That foundation is your lifestyle—diet, exercise, stress management, sleep, and vitamin R.

You may think, "Yeah, I know I should eat better," or "Yeah, I know I should exercise more."

Or you may be that woman who says, "These changes are too much…it's too hard…I can't do it." Or, "I'm too tired to exercise. Plus my brain is mush by noon." And if you cannot sleep, "How do you expect me to sleep better if I don't get rid of these damn night sweats?"

You may think that what I'm going to suggest is pie in the sky—too good to be true—because it's such simple advice that it cannot possibly work. But, it does. Most every time. With most every patient.

Are you really ready to get started? Are you really ready to fix your fatigue?

One more thing before we move forward.

This can be very overwhelming; nobody likes to change. (Not even me!) So my suggestion for you is to just try it. Start today, and begin to master only one thing—whichever aspect of your lifestyle you want, whether diet, exercise, stress management, sleep, or vitamin R. (But I will tell you that what you put into your mouth will most likely have the biggest impact on how you feel.)

When you master one area of your lifestyle, then move on to another. Just take it step by step.

Consider this: Let's say you get only 10 percent better from each area of your lifestyle that you work on. You will not feel any different by making one or two changes. But do them all, and you are looking at a 50 percent improvement at least, and that you *will* feel.

Your long-term energy awaits!

Diet—Let Your Food Be Your Medicine

Food can be your medicine, or it can be your poison. Let's make it your medicine!

You probably think it's impossible to change your diet. I'm living proof that it's not. You *can* do it. Trust me—if I can do it, so can you, especially if you follow my guidelines.

Here's what most women eat that keeps them in fatigue:

- ➢ too many carbs
- ➢ too much sugar
- ➢ not enough healthy fats
- ➢ not enough protein and fiber
- ➢ foods you are allergic or sensitive to (knowingly or unknowingly)

Here's *how* most women eat that keeps them in fatigue:

- ➢ eating a lousy breakfast or skipping breakfast altogether
- ➢ skipping other meals

To get out of fatigue you need to:

- ➢ stop the carbs
- ➢ reduce sugar significantly
- ➢ add in more healthy fats
- ➢ eat enough protein
- ➢ eat enough fiber
- ➢ remove foods you are allergic or sensitive to
- ➢ definitely eat a good breakfast
- ➢ eat three meals a day plus two snacks
- ➢ eat every two to three hours

I know, I know—this sounds near impossible. But it isn't.

There is one diet that meets all of these guidelines and still lets you eat plenty of delicious foods. It is the Paleo Diet.

The Paleo Diet

Now, I can't take credit for the Paleo Diet. It's the brainchild of Loren Cordain, PhD. The Paleo Diet is basically eating like our ancestors did. Like a caveman.

See, we have modified and hybridized and frankensized our foods much faster than our bodies have been able to keep up with. Because of this, we are in general seeing more fatigue, hormonal problems, digestive problems, allergies, autoimmune disease, and more.

Foods Highest in Fiber *and* **Paleo-Diet Friendly**
➤ sweet potato ➤ avocado ➤ berries ➤ pear ➤ mango ➤ apple ➤ coconut ➤ leafy greens ➤ broccoli
Aim for 30-60 grams of fiber daily. Make sure to drink plenty of water with your fiber or you may get constipated.

Remember when you were a kid? How many of the kids in your class had a peanut allergy? Or, any allergy to any food?

Today food allergy is *so* common that people think it's normal— which it isn't!

So the Paleo Diet helps get us back to the basic diet we ate long ago, before we started screwing up the food supply. It's basically meat and fish (protein), veggies, fruits, nuts, seeds, and healthy fats.

It doesn't contain wheat or other grains, gluten, sugar, dairy, legumes/beans, or unhealthy fats.

I know what you're saying right now—"What the heck CAN I eat?"

☞ Imagine your plate. Fill half with veggies. On the other half, fill one corner with protein (meat, fish)—about the size of your palm. In the area that remains, add a serving of fruit, and a bit of healthy fat (avocado is a good choice, as are raw nuts). That is a Paleo plate.

The Paleo Diet is your perfect ticket out of food-choice-induced fatigue.

What I love about the Paleo Diet is that it removes *all* the stuff that promotes fatigue. Harmful inflammatory foods are gone: grains, dairy, and legumes. Most of the common food allergies are gone: wheat, gluten, dairy, and soy. And you get nutrients, antioxidants, fiber, and healthy fat.

Warning: I actually *don't* recommend you jump headfirst into the Paleo Diet. Most women end up overwhelmed and quit within days. I don't want you to be a quitter. I want you to be successful with this so you can fix your fatigue.

Here's what worked for me when I was changing my diet, and it is the key to success: Work on one meal at a time, and only one meal at a time. Period.

Start with breakfast. Work on that, and only that. Do an Internet search on "Paleo breakfast." There are plenty of ideas and recipes online. Search online for "Paleo smoothies" or "fast Paleo breakfast" to get ideas for those days when you need to make breakfast at lightning speed.

It may take a few weeks to really feel like you've mastered that one meal. That's okay!

Once you get to the point where you've mastered Paleo breakfast, then move on to lunch and transition lunch over to Paleo.

And, once you master lunch, then do Paleo snacks, and lastly Paleo dinner. It will take a few months to really master the entire routine of a Paleo Diet, and that's fine!

(Remember, the tortoise won the race!)

Easy Paleo Breakfast Ideas

I've found that Paleo breakfast can be the most difficult for patients to wrap their heads around. There are a lot of choices—more than you think!

Eggs
Unless you have a sensitivity to them, eggs are great and can be eaten every day, despite what you've been told about your cholesterol. Try an omelet with lots of veggies inside, or make yourself a frittata with lots of veggies, and a side of fruit (do not exceed two servings of fruit daily though).

Don't have time for that? Hardboiled eggs are a good choice. Hard boil them on the weekend—a full dozen or two—then crack and eat on the run.

Smoothie

Even easier is a smoothie. A NutriBullet blender works great for this and comes with a terrific recipe book.

Stuff your NutriBullet (or other blender) with two a big handfuls of greens (spinach is a good one to start with, and you won't even taste it, I swear!). Then add in a cup of berries (I like blueberries because they're considered a superfood and they're low on the glycemic index).

Top it off with a spoonful of flaxseed powder, a spoonful of chia seeds, a small handful of nuts, and some avocado to give it a smooth, creamy texture (plus it adds more fiber and healthy fat too).

Add coconut water (it's high in electrolytes, especially potassium), and blitz until smooth. That's my Dr. Carri's Easy Paleo Smoothie. (I can hear it now—"He likes it! He likes it! Mikey likes it!")

It would be ideal to be 100 percent on the Paleo Diet, but believe me—I'm a realist. Most women can't do 100 percent. So, strive for Paleo 80 percent of the time, and 20 percent of the time you can cheat. That translates into one full day per week (three meals) off the Paleo Diet.

If you're in need of an extreme energy transformation, work toward 100 percent Paleo to achieve the fastest rise in your energy.

You will be amazed at how good you feel on the Paleo Diet. Now, I'm not saying you'll have to stay on the Paleo Diet for the rest of your life…just long enough for your body chemistry to really get back into balance. Once that happens, you can make the choice whether you want to stay on the Paleo Diet or go back to your old diet.

With a quick Internet search, you will find thousands of Web pages, blogs, and videos, all for free, to help you switch over to a Paleo Diet.

Blood Sugar and the Paleo Diet

The Paleo Diet is especially great for women who suffer from blood sugar problems—low blood sugar, high blood sugar, insulin resistance, even diabetes. To know what your blood sugar is doing, there are two things you can check for, and I recommend you do both.

One is to take the questionnaire (if you didn't earlier):

Hypoglycemia Questionnaire	Yes	No
I crave sweets, especially during the day.		
I get cranky if I miss a meal.		
I depend on coffee to get myself started and/or to keep myself going.		
I get lightheaded if I miss a meal.		
Eating relieves my fatigue.		
I feel shaky if I wait too long to eat.		
I feel agitated, easily upset, nervous between meals.		
I have a poor memory and am forgetful.		

If you have three or more "yes" answers, you are more prone to having low blood sugar, or hypoglycemia. This is easily remedied with the Paleo Diet.

The second is to check your A1C. (See Chapter 5: Blood Sugar Imbalance.)

If you're on insulin or insulin-controlling medications, note that as the Paleo Diet fixes your blood sugar, you will need less and less medication. I've even have patients get off their medications completely once the underlying causes have been addressed.

Note: Don't try to manipulate your medication levels on your own. That's what the professionals are for, so consult your prescribing doctor.

**Liz's Fatigue Journey—
Now I Actually Feel BETTER Than My Old Self!!!**

Dr. Carri: Liz! Thanks for meeting with me to share your fatigue story with our readers. I'm sure there is a woman out there who is going to read your story and resonate with it. You're going to change her life!

Tell me about your fatigue. How long did you have it? What treatment did you try? What doctors did you see?

Liz: It's been many, many years that I've been dealing with fatigue. Maybe close to fourteen years—a long time! When it first started, there was a lot happening in my personal life and at the office. A lot of stress. And then fatigue started slowly taking over my life. I had many sleepless nights. I would sleep maybe two to four hours. Some nights I wouldn't sleep at all. It wasn't like that every night, but it happened a lot.

I tried medications. One of them was lorazepam (Ativan). It worked at the beginning, but that didn't last long. Then it stopped working altogether.

And I tried all kinds of sleeping pills. All kinds! Most of them didn't work for me consistently. I also tried a lot of natural stuff. It didn't work either. I would go to the health food store, and they would say "try this" or "try that." But most you shouldn't mix with medications, so then I was in a bind. I saw my family doctor, and a psychiatrist, and a naturopath. Nothing worked.

Dr. Carri: What was your life like back when you had fatigue?

Liz: It was very bad! It was hard to concentrate. It was hard to have a full day's work, and that's when I had a full-time job. I was a boss and had employees under me, and that was very stressful. Plus we had a business, so I was working full-time during the day at my job and then worked at our business on nights and weekends. I did that for five years. At the end of five years, I couldn't deal with it anymore. Then the divorce happened. Everything happened at the same time, so it was very, very stressful.

Dr. Carri: That was like a sixty-hour work week for five years?

Liz: Or more! I worked Friday night, Saturday, Sunday, plus two or three nights during the week, plus my full-time job. It was way too much.

Dr. Carri: Did you have any other symptoms besides the fatigue that you were really struggling with? You mentioned difficulty sleeping.

Liz: Yes, difficulty sleeping. Plus, I was perimenopausal and I was hemorrhaging often. I guess the hormones were imbalanced, and I was too stressed. I didn't know what was going on really.

I had a D&C, and then another, and another, and another. But I kept hemorrhaging. Then the doctor was talking about a hysterectomy. I didn't want that because I knew the underlying cause was all the stress and my lifestyle. If I could have dealt with that back then, I wouldn't have needed a hysterectomy.

Family, friends, a lot of people were telling me, "You should follow your doctor's advice and get the hysterectomy. You'll have no more problems, and blah, blah, blah." But I didn't want that. I knew that when you do that you're losing part of your body, which is there to help you. It's there for a reason. I knew I didn't want to go that route.

Dr. Carri: Plus it doesn't actually fix the underlying hormonal imbalance either. It's just another Band-Aid. It's a pretty permanent Band-Aid.

Liz: I started perimenopause when I was thirty-six years old! The stress didn't help!

Dr. Carri: These days it's actually not unusual for perimenopause to start in women's thirties. Mainly it's due to our stressful lifestyles. Was there anything about having fatigue that had you really worried or afraid or angry?

Liz: When you're fatigued and stressed, you lose your joie de vivre. Life isn't fun anymore. It was hard to concentrate. My work had to be double and triple checked. I lost confidence in myself because I was so stressed. I was wondering what the hell was going on with me. Plus with the medications I tried— antidepressants—I tried quite a few before we found the correct one, and that was stressful because of all the side effects.

I was gaining weight. I was getting anxiety attacks. And some of them gave me migraines. Upset stomach—I wasn't digesting well. So the appetite with the digestion and the food I was eating, even though it was healthy food and lots of veggies and stuff like that, it wasn't working. I had to buy new clothes. It was frustrating!

Dr. Carri: After you met with me, what was it that finally made you decide to go ahead with the treatment program that I put together for you?

Liz: I knew I had nothing to lose. The doctors weren't helping me except for handing me prescriptions. So I thought, "Let's try this and see if it works."

Before I started with you, my sleep was terrible. I would go two or three days in a row where I wasn't sleeping at all. You had me do a saliva test for cortisol and melatonin. You found my cortisol was too high at night, and my melatonin was too low at night. *(Liz's melatonin was 1.1 pg/ml. Normal is 12.0-23.0 pg/ml.)* No wonder I couldn't sleep!

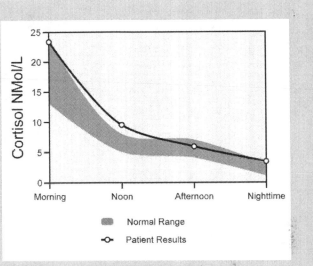

Liz's cortisol test results

You recommended specific supplements for me—vitamins, herbs, and amino acids—and that first night, my God, I slept like a baby! I slept eight hours! And I've been sleeping every night since!

Dr. Carri: Once we were able to get you sleeping, I knew the next step was to tackle your diet and let your food be your medicine. I recommended a book called *The Plan*. I wanted to see which foods were your friends and which were your enemies. Eating the wrong foods will only promote fatigue, weight gain, chronic pain, and hormonal imbalance. So when I first recommended *The Plan*, what did you think about that?

Liz: Well, I felt like it was something that I could try. I went and bought the book. Read it. Then I said, "Okay, I'll try it." It was really hard to follow and do precisely, but I did it. It took four or five weeks. That's when I noticed which foods were my enemies. I found fourteen foods that were my enemies. And when I eliminated those foods from my diet, I felt better, I felt stronger, the foggy brain left. It made quite a difference! Plus sleeping better. There were major, major changes!

Dr. Carri: I remember you also mentioning pain. Let's talk about the chronic pain that you suffered with for so many years.

Liz: I was seeing the chiropractor two or three times a week. It was pretty bad! Neck pain. Back pain. Pain in my shoulders. But as I started with *The Plan* and I started working with you, it's been five or six weeks since my last adjustment, and I feel really good! My pain is gone!

In the book it says food sensitivities will get your body inflamed and will make you hurt, and that was me! And my chiropractor always had a hard time adjusting me too. At my last visit he said, "What have you been doing? Your back feels great! It's so easy to adjust you. What have you been doing?" I said, "I've been seeing your neighbor next door—the naturopath!" (Laughs.)

Dr. Carri: Liz, when I start talking to patients about food and food sensitivities and changing their diet, with a lot of them I can see it in their eyes—they glaze right over with fear. And some of them don't even believe me, I can tell. They don't believe that food can be *that* powerful! That's why I wanted to have your story for this book!

Liz: Food *is* medicine, so they should at least try. Read *The Plan* and try it! It's amazing how you feel afterward! My fatigue is GONE! My pain is GONE! My digestive problems are GONE!

My foggy brain is GONE! I actually feel BETTER than my old self!!!

Dr. Carri: What is life like now that you're better? What can you do now that you couldn't do before?

Liz: I've started walking again. Exercising. I have energy to declutter my house. That's a big project for me. A lot of stuff piles up when you have fatigue for so long!

I'm trying new recipes, and cooking is fun again for a change. I'm into cookbooks, and I'm trying this and I'm trying that, and it's fun!

And I have more energy! And I've got more joie de vivre!! And I feel happy!!!

I live in a condo. People in the building, strangers I know only because they also live in my building, have seen me now and said, "You look younger!" I reply, "Well, thank you, because I know I'm not getting any younger!"

Dr. Carri: That's fantastic! What do you see your life like in the future now that your energy is back?

Liz: I'm getting my house organized. And I'm working on opening a business. I want to travel. I want to go out with friends and enjoy life! It's been quite a ride!

Dr. Carri: Do you have any advice for other women struggling with fatigue?

Liz: The first thing is to have their saliva test done. Look over everything and see what should be dealt with first. Then check for food sensitivities and deal with those, even if it takes two or three months. By eliminating one food, and the next, and the next, they'll feel much, much better!

And thank you, Dr. Carri, for helping me! For going the correct route, knowing what to do, and running the right tests—because that was a big thing! Everything is connected, but it can be such a big mess when you feel the way I did!

Dr. Carri: It's not always easy to figure out the mess. But, like I say: Find the cause. Fix the cause. Feel normal again! That's the power of functional medicine. Thank you, Liz!

Chronic Low-Grade Inflammation—How It Relates to Fatigue and Your Diet

All the researchers are talking about it these days—inflammation.

What is inflammation exactly? Think about if you sprained your ankle. What would you notice? Swelling, redness, pain, heat. These are the four cardinal signs of inflammation.

But what does that have to do with fatigue?

The more inflammation you have, the more cortisol your body produces, at the expense of the hormones. You end up with hormonal imbalance, often including thyroid imbalance. That leads to fatigue.

Maybe you've heard that researchers are finding chronic low-grade inflammation to be the underlying reason for so many of today's chronic diseases. Like arthritis, osteoporosis, obesity, heart disease, and diabetes.

More inflammation equals more fatigue.

Want to stop your fatigue fast? Ditch the inflammatory foods.

Inflammatory foods are:

> ➢ sugar
> ➢ carbs
> ➢ grains
> ➢ alcohol (okay, a little bit of red wine is allowed)
> ➢ legumes
> ➢ dairy
> ➢ meat that is not organic grass fed
> ➢ and any foods you are allergic to

Reduce your chronic low-grade inflammation, and you'll increase your energy!

The Dirty Dozen Plus—Foods you should ***always buy certified organic*** because the non-organics have the <u>highest</u> levels of pesticides (from the Environmental Working Group, www.EWG.org).	The Clean Fifteen—Foods you don't need to buy certified organic because they have the <u>lowest</u> levels of pesticides (from the Environmental Working Group, www.EWG.org).
1. apples	1. asparagus
2. celery	2. avocados
3. cherry tomatoes	3. cabbage
4. cucumbers	4. cantaloupe
5. grapes	5. sweet corn
6. hot peppers	6. eggplant
7. nectarines (imported)	7. grapefruit
8. peaches	8. kiwi
9. potatoes	9. mangos
10. spinach	10. mushrooms
11. strawberries	11. onions
12. bell peppers	12. papayas
13. kale/collard greens	13. pineapple
14. zucchini/summer squash	14. sweet peas (frozen)
	15. sweet potatoes

Diet—Drink & Hydration

What you drink is just as important as what you eat. Let's face it—most women are dehydrated. They just don't drink enough water.

A Solution for Incontinence

Now for some women, dehydration is because of urinary incontinence. They have a hard time holding in their urine and tend to dribble, so they just stop drinking water to avoid the mess and potential embarrassment.

You've probably been told to expect to be urine incontinent after having babies, or to expect to be incontinent when you hit menopause. To expect that every time you sneeze, or cough, or laugh that a little bit of urine will leak out.

Ladies, this is never normal!

If you have any amount of urine incontinence, I urge you to see a physiotherapist/physical therapist who specializes in pelvic floor problems. This is a specialty within the field of physical therapy, so make sure your therapist is trained properly.

It is quite an intimate ordeal, kind of like getting a pap smear. The therapist will put you in the stirrups and manually assess the muscles throughout your pelvic floor. They will be feeling for muscles that are too tight, muscles that are too loose, and knots in your muscles. Again, all of this is done with a hands-on approach. Not with biofeedback. Not with electrodes.

Most women with urine incontinence have been told to do Kegel exercises. Well, if nobody checks to see if you're doing Kegels properly, then how do you know if you're even doing them the right way? And, if your pelvic floor muscles are already too tight, those Kegels won't even work! (Most women have pelvic floor muscles that are actually too tight, so Kegels are useless.)

To find a physiotherapist/physical therapist trained in the specialty of pelvic floor rehabilitation, please refer to the Resources section.

Water

What *is* the right amount of water to be drinking?

Half your ideal body weight (in pounds) as ounces of water every day. For example, if your ideal body weight is 150 pounds, then you should be drinking 150 divided by 2 equals 75 ounces of fluid every day. One cup is 8 ounces, so roughly 7½ cups of water.

Any water is better than no water, but preferred is filtered alkaline water.

You can also get your water from drinking herbal teas. Drink them hot. Drink them cold. I don't care. Just drink them. I especially like passionflower tea cold. Green tea and hibiscus are excellent choices as well. They have many healthy properties. Try to drink two cups of green tea every day purely for the health benefits, as green tea is considered a superfood. Again, hot or cold—it doesn't matter.

If you've never had green tea before, go out and try a bunch of different varieties to find one you like. If you don't usually care for green tea, go out and find one you like. There is one out there with your name on it! I personally can't stand plain green tea, so I buy a variety that also has peppermint leaves mixed in, or even lemongrass and ginger. The green tea taste gets lost in the background of the other herbs.

Lastly, tea can be loaded with pesticides, so use certified organic herbal tea.

Alcohol

Alcohol adds to fatigue because it fuels cortisol imbalance, thereby robbing you of sex hormones and stressing your thyroid hormone levels. Come on, ladies, most of you already know it's bad anyways.

Should you stop drinking alcohol? That's a no-brainer: yes.

If you want the quickest results from this program, you need to cut out 100 percent of the alcohol from your diet for six months. The faster you do it, the faster you'll feel more energized.

Does this mean you can never drink alcohol again? No. Eventually, as you work your way through my program, you'll find what your body can tolerate.

A little red wine is healthy.

Just a little, though.

Caffeine

Caffeine, like alcohol, fuels cortisol imbalance, thereby robbing you of sex hormones and stressing your thyroid gland. It's best to cut out all caffeine during this program to get the fastest energy replenishment and the most long-lasting results.

Be careful with cutting out caffeine, though. It's a major addiction for a lot of women. You'll go through caffeine withdrawal if you don't take it out of your diet slowly.

Don't think that decaf is safe either. Decaf always has a certain amount of caffeine still intact, and this level varies from company to company. Just avoid decaf all together.

I know most of you rely on caffeine to simply get through your day. Without it you would be useless. I get that. So what I recommend is that you save this step for last. Do everything else I mention in Part 2 of this book first to build your health back up. Then, by the time you cut out the caffeine, it will be easier to survive without it. You won't need to rely on the energy from caffeine. Your body will be producing abundant energy all on its own.

Hint: If you're the type of person who is very sensitive to caffeine and/or alcohol, you probably have an underlying imbalance within your liver detoxification pathways that needs to be addressed. Your functional medicine doctor can help you with this.

With these updates to your eating and drinking habits, you will soon feel your energy returning!

Chapter 11

Exercise to Enjoy Abundant Energy

Exercise and Metabolism

When it comes to exercise, more is not necessarily better.

If your metabolism is broken, the more exercise you do will actually further damage your metabolism, and the more fatigue you will feel.

You may be this person, or you may know this person: Despite eating fewer and fewer calories and exercising like a madwoman, your weight does not budge. This is because your metabolism is damaged. Always make sure you're getting balanced exercise— equal amounts of stretching, cardio, and resistance in your week— to help rebalance your metabolism.

Many women rely almost exclusively on cardio for fat burning. This doesn't work! You need to balance that cardio with stretching and resistance exercises.

I find that many women shy away from resistance exercise. Resistance means weight lifting of some form—actual weights (dumbbells, barbells) or body weight. Women tell me they're afraid they will get too muscly. Ladies, it simply will not happen! You will not get overly muscly unless you solely do resistance exercise, and a lot of it!

Again, the key is balance between stretching, cardio, and resistance.

Exercise should give you energy. If you feel really tired after exercising, you did too much! I've had some patients whose metabolism is so broken that even ten minutes of exercise gets them dog tired. It's just too much for their metabolism to handle. I tell them to cut back to six minutes, or even four minutes. However many minutes you can tolerate and still feel good after, then stick to that level until you get stronger and can do more. Take it slow. There's no rush.

In functional medicine we are better able to guide your "personal exercise prescription" once we know what your cortisol is doing— if it's too high, too low, or on a roller coaster.

Could You Have a Mitochondrial Imbalance?

If you're doing all the right things but you're still dog tired after exercising, consider you may have a mitochondrial imbalance. Mitochondrial imbalance (or dysfunctional mitochondria) is part of my Expanded Fatigue List, so if that description fits you, you can learn more by getting a free copy of my Expanded List via the Special Bonus section at the end of this book.

Beautiful Benefits of Exercise

In addition to increased energy and fitness, here are six more beautiful benefits of exercise:

- ➢ boosts brain function
- ➢ prevents decline in memory
- ➢ improves nutrient-absorbing digestion

➢ alleviates anxiety and depression
➢ increases relaxation
➢ improves sleep

Better energy, better body, better mind. Long-term. That's worth getting pumped about!

Chapter 12

Sensational Sleep

Identify Sleep Disturbers

It almost goes without saying that in order to help treat fatigue, you need to make sure you're getting a good night's rest.

There are multiple reasons why women do not sleep well.

Blood Sugar

Sometimes the blood sugar dips down too low at night, and this triggers you to wake up. A small protein snack before bed can help resolve this.

Cortisol

Sometimes the cortisol is too high at night, and this makes it hard to fall asleep and/or stay asleep. Saliva cortisol testing can tell you if this is true for your case. And even if you don't know your cortisol level, following all the steps in Part 2 of this book, "Build Your Foundation for *Lasting* Energy," will help your cortisol overall anyway.

Melatonin

Some women don't produce enough melatonin. Melatonin is the sleep hormone made by the pineal gland in the brain. The pineal gland makes melatonin when it gets dark, and stops making melatonin when it gets light.

LOW MELATONIN DUE TO BRIGHT LIGHT

You may not produce adequate melatonin simply because you're exposed to bright light for far too long into the evening. Bright light from television screens. Bright light from computer screens, tablets, and iPhones—these are worse than televisions because they're actually brighter than television screens.

The remedy for this is to stop all computer, tablet, iPhone, and television use two hours before bedtime.

Use dimmers on your lights, and two hours before bed, dim the lights. Read a relaxing book, something that doesn't require a lot of thinking, such as light fiction. You might like to knit or crochet. You can do your journaling here.

Anything you can think of that does not require bright light or brain power, that's what you should be doing at bedtime.

LOW MELATONIN DUE TO LOW SEROTONIN

Melatonin is made from serotonin. When women do not produce adequate melatonin, it makes me wonder, "Why? Are they not making enough serotonin either?"

The biggest source of serotonin production is the digestive tract. The digestive tract is responsible for upwards of 90 percent of the serotonin production for your body.

Oftentimes, poor sleep is a sign of low melatonin, which is because of low serotonin production, which is actually due to an underlying digestive problem. Like a chronic infection, food allergies, or leaky gut syndrome.

Many doctors will recommend melatonin for sleeping, and taking melatonin supplements can be helpful, but be aware that this is only a Band-Aid solution. You always want to find and fix the underlying cause.

Melatonin can be measured with a saliva test, and from there a functional medicine doctor can help you find and fix the underlying cause.

Find the cause. Fix the cause. Feel normal again!

Sleep "Hygiene"

Sleep "hygiene" is a term we use to describe the necessary factors for promoting good sleep. You've heard of oral hygiene—the necessary factors to promote good oral health, like brushing and flossing regularly. Well, there's sleep hygiene too.

Good Night, Light!

One of the easiest tools I have found to improve quality of sleep across the board (and I do this myself) is a simple eye mask.

This will often give you deeper, more restful sleep because it blocks out *all* light. Even small amounts of light from alarm clocks can blunt melatonin production and affect your sleep.

If the eye mask works for you, then it's time to block out all sources of light in your bedroom. Your bedroom should really be like a cave. You shouldn't even be able to see your hand in front of your face—that's how dark your bedroom should be. If you can still see your hand, your room isn't dark enough.

I personally got my wake-up call on this (☺) when I went on a cruise. My room was an inside cabin, so there were no windows. This really freaked me out. All the other cruises I'd been on always had a balcony or a window…an "escape" route (I think I've watched the movie *Titanic* too many times).

To me the inside cabin was claustrophobic—until that first night I went to sleep. I remember there was light spilling into the room underneath the cabin door, so I stuffed a towel under the door to block the light. Once I did this, the room went completely black, like a cave. I had to be careful not to break a toe on the furniture.

And you know what? My husband and I both slept like babies! Every night we had deep, refreshing sleep. From that day forward, I knew how important it was to sleep in cave-like darkness.

So block out all sources of light from your bedroom. Light creeps in around window shades and blinds. Stop this with better blinds and drapes, or use the Blackout EZ Window Cover system for this (see the Resources section).

We get light from alarm clocks, phones…pretty much anything electrical these days will cast some sort of light. I recommend taking all unnecessary light-emitting electronics out of the room completely, or cover up the lights completely before you go to bed every night. It will be worth it.

A Restful Routine

Establish a sleep routine. Go to bed at the same time every night (including weekends), and wake up at the same time every day (including weekends). Stick to this schedule to maintain good, steady REM cycles that enable you to wake up feeling rested and energized.

Marvelous Mattresses

On that same cruise that I talked about earlier, the other big reason I got such great sleep was because of the fantastic bedding. It was like sleeping on a cloud.

Consider investing in better bedding—feather bed, feather duvet, feather pillows...even a new mattress. You spend a third of your life sleeping. Invest in your happiness! You're worth it!

Still More Slumber Secrets

Remember: no alcohol or caffeine in the evening, and no exercise after seven at night, as these interfere with quality of sleep.

Have a cup of herbal tea, like chamomile tea, before bed.

Keep a note pad beside your bed. Don't try to remember everything! Clear out your head; write it all down before bed.

Also, count your blessings—do a gratitude journal. List five things, no matter how big or small, that you are grateful for. Forgive yourself and others for any hurts accumulated through the day.

Lastly, use one or two drops of lavender oil on your pillow.

It will all help you sleep better. And the faster you start sleeping better, the faster your fatigue will stop.

Sleep, like food and water, is a necessity for good health. While you sleep your body is actually very active detoxifying, repairing, and rebuilding.

For women who have not been getting good sleep: Once your sleep mechanism kicks back in, your body will need to stock up on sleep. Don't be surprised if you need an unusual amount of sleep for a while. This is your body getting out of sleep debt.

Anne's Fatigue Journey— Fatigue So Bad That She Slept through a Two-Week Vacation

Dr. Carri: Anne, thank you for being so kind as to share your story with everyone!

Anne: You're welcome! It's my pleasure!

Dr. Carri: We're doing this interview to help other women out there struggling with fatigue. Women feeling just like you used to feel. Let's give them some hope and show them it *is* possible to fix their fatigue. Anne, tell us about your fatigue.

Anne: Well, when you have fatigue so bad that you come to a point when the thought of dying in the prime of your life doesn't sound like such a bad thing, and would even give you relief, that's kind of sad. I had these thoughts often, though.

I work full time as a nurse. I would work eight hours, go home, then sleep for a couple hours, get up, putter around for a couple hours, go back to bed, and wake up the next day just as tired as before.

I was angry at having to go through this. Doing it over and over again, day after day, was pretty depressing. I've done the same work for years, and it shouldn't be a struggle, except it was!

I lost my sense of humor. I felt just awful. I couldn't think of anything to laugh about. I was angry all the time, and so tired. I had a hard time coping with people in general. Everything was overwhelming. I had to check everything three or four times to make sure I didn't make any mistakes at work.

Dr. Carri: Because your brain wasn't working very well? Poor memory? Foggy brain?

Anne: Poor memory, yes! I thought I was starting to have dementia, and I'm only fifty-one! On top of that, I had migraines. It was upsetting not being able to enjoy life, even my time off.

I did see my family doctor many times. He's helped me a great deal. But being on an antidepressant never felt like a real solution for my fatigue. He was very supportive, but there was a limit to what he could do to help me.

I was always *so* tired. I wondered if I had sleep apnea. I was sent for a sleep study, and the results said everything was normal. I also asked for a full cardiac workup to see if I had my father's genes. I didn't want to have a heart attack at age sixty like he did. I was just so tired that I thought, "I must be *really* ill!"

Dr. Carri: And the cardiac tests were normal?

Anne: Yes, everything was normal. Basically what pushed me to finally call you, Dr. Carri, is I took a vacation and slept for two weeks. Then I felt okay for about a week at work. But then the fatigue was right back to where I was before the vacation!

Dr. Carri: So, you've been struggling with fatigue for about forty years?

Anne: Yes. On and off.

Dr. Carri: And your family doctor called it depression?

Anne: Yes. He was very good at listening to my complaints, and ran blood tests every year. I'm low in iron, so I would take an iron supplement, but my fatigue still continued.

I took antidepressants on and off, but I didn't want to. It wasn't solving whatever was wrong with me. But that's all that he could offer. Could I have pushed for more? I don't know. I do know that I didn't get what I thought I really needed—to find the underlying cause of my fatigue.

Dr. Carri: At that point, did you think that you really had depression? Or, do you think you had depression and something else going on? Or, did you think this was all something else completely, and not actually depression?

Anne: That's it! I didn't really know! I said, "Okay, the doctor thinks that I have depression, so it must be that," and I would see people every day at work on antidepressants, because it's supposed to be a "fix all." But I didn't want those chemicals in my body.

Dr. Carri: Then you called my office. We sat down for our first visit, and then we got copies of all your past blood work to start looking for clues to the underlying cause of your fatigue.

All I found was that your B12 was low. Just so you know, your family doctor was very thorough with your blood work. I don't see that in most cases, so you have a great family doctor!

For your case, I knew there was more going on, and I had a gut feeling that we had to treat both your adrenals and your brain at the same time. I don't usually do that with patients, because it can get quite expensive with all the testing and supplements to take—it's a lot of pills to swallow; I know from personal experience! I forewarned you about all that, but you were a real trooper and decided to just go for it!

I did a saliva test and saw your cortisol was at Stage 2 Adrenal Fatigue, so we started treatment for that.

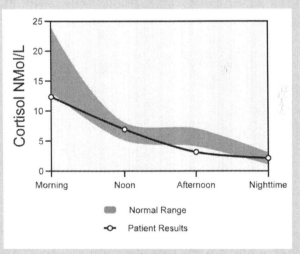

Anne's cortisol test results

I also had you start a Brain Balancing Program. Again, you're one of the few patients that I've been that aggressive with—treating both cortisol and brain at the same time.

That's part of the reason I was hoping you would share your story with us, because it took guts and courage to follow through with all my recommendations. I know that it was sometimes hard and overwhelming, but look at you now!

Anne: Yes, I was *very* ready to try it. I said, "Enough is enough!" The moodiness, sleeping my vacations away, struggling to go to work. Within two weeks on the program, I started seeing some changes. After a month, I knew I was definitely better. And after six weeks, I was feeling so much better!

Dr. Carri: I'm looking through your file. Within a month, your energy went from a two out of ten to a five out of ten!

Next I asked you to try the Paleo Diet, which you did, and you said, "Holy Paleo!" because your energy then shot up to eight out of ten! Plus, you started to lose weight and your migraines stopped.

Anne: Yes! And my sense of humor came back! I can laugh things off. I can just move on. I can joke with people. I don't get angry. It has helped with all that, and helped me communicate better. My self-esteem is back. I have confidence again!

Dr. Carri: You've said that you used to be so angry inside. That's a side of you that I've never seen, and I wouldn't have even guessed that you had that anger inside. It's so great that you feel like your normal self, happy and smiley!

Anne: Yes! I can enjoy my friends and family now. I can actually go back home and pick up the phone and call people.

Before, all I could think of was to go home and sleep and hide in my cave like a bear.

Dr. Carri: Are you exercising again?

Anne: Well I'm not right now, but I went to Mexico for two weeks and I had so much fun, and had so much energy—I loved it! And I came back rested! I didn't sleep my vacation away. I've got pictures to prove it! My friend and I are planning to fully renovate an old mill and eventually start a bed and breakfast.

Dr. Carri: That's amazing! I didn't even know any of that. How exciting! And that's a big project!

Anne: It is a big project. I feel like I can tackle it now.

Dr. Carri: There are a lot of details just renovating, plus running the business! Wow! Good for you. Let me know when it's ready for guests!

Anne, one last question for our readers. What advice do you have for other women struggling with fatigue?

Anne: Just do it! Go see Dr. Carri! She understood me and believed me when I told her how I was feeling. She ran tests my doctor didn't know to run, and found the real underlying problems. Dr. Carri had me take all kinds of vitamins and change my diet. I was very overwhelmed at first, but I decided to let go of some things in my life that weren't important so I could focus on my health. Dr. Carri was my cheerleader and gave me the answers I had been looking for!

Dr. Carri: Anything else you want to add for our readers?

Anne: Have hope! Be good to yourself. Concentrate on what is really important—your health! It isn't cheap to see Dr. Carri, but the expense has been totally worth it for me!

Chapter 13

Vitamin R—Rest, Relaxation, Recreation!

Rest. Relaxation. Recreation. I like to call it vitamin R.

What do *you* do for rest, relaxation, and recreation? Most of us have been conditioned to "do, do, do," and we forget to "rest, rest, rest."

The "do, do, do" causes the hormone cortisol to get out of balance, and this—as you probably know by now—is the number one reason most women are fatigued. When you get more vitamin R in your life, your cortisol levels should become more normal. So give yourself permission to rest, relax, and have fun!

Take that vacation you've always dreamed about. Get back to that hobby that got put on the back burner all those years ago. Do something every day that brings you joy. Consider it doctor's orders!

Stress Management—Body Chemistry Effects and Solutions

Fatigue is the third most common symptom of stress. Chronic stress causes cortisol to get out of balance, and cortisol is what is keeping most women in fatigue.

First the stress creates cortisol imbalance, which then has a domino effect and robs you of DHEA, estrogen, progesterone, testosterone, and thyroid hormones.

Stress is not only mental and emotional stress either. There's also physical stressors. Eating an unhealthy diet creates stress on your body. Eating food you are allergic to creates stress to your body. Chronic inflammation is a stress to your body. Toxins stress your body, as well as hidden infections. Estrogen surges stress your body too.

When we deal with stress, we need to deal with all the physical causes, and also the between-your-two-ears mental and emotional causes. Give yourself permission to talk to a therapist if needed. Talking to a good friend will also help a lot.

As you have seen me write over and over again, find the underlying cause, then fix the underlying cause. Then, and only then, will you fix your fatigue and feel normal again.

Deep Breathing

Want a guaranteed way to relax? Do some deep breathing. It always works.

Try it right now. Take a deep breath in, all the way down into your belly. Hold it for three seconds, and then slowly exhale. Repeat this five times.

I can already see the stress melting off you.

Do some deep breathing periodically throughout your day. I know women who actually schedule it into their day. Stick it into your electronic calendar with a reminder to take a break and breathe. Or use an old fashioned sticky note reminder.

Deep breathing works especially well when you're in the moment of feeling stressed. Like when you're sitting in traffic. Or when you come home and the kids have made a mess of the house. Or when your spouse is driving you crazy. Or when the boss puts another project on your already full to-do list.

Breathe.

Meditation

Meditation is a classic way to increase your vitamin R. If you're like me, you get very frustrated with meditation quickly. But what I've learned is to meditate in small amounts. Like any form of exercise, if you try to do too much too soon you will likely fail. So start with just five minutes a day.

There are many different types of meditation available. A quick Internet search will give you many Web pages, blogs, and videos to choose from. There are even free courses available, locally in your community, and online.

Personally, I'm the type of person who does better with a scheduled course. It helps keep me accountable. I don't want to let my instructor down. Plus, forking out some cold hard cash helps too. I want to get my money's worth, so I don't miss a class!

Two Meditation Samples

There are two types of meditation that work best for me, so I'll share them with you. The first one I call Four Square Breathing.

FOUR SQUARE BREATHING

You close your eyes and imagine a square. Inhale as you mentally follow one side of the square to the corner. When you get to the corner in your mind, hold your breath for a count of five seconds, and then slowly exhale. As you exhale, follow the next side of the square to the next corner.

When you get to the next corner, hold your exhale for a count of five seconds, and then slowly inhale again, following the square to the next corner.

The other meditation that really works for me I call Color Breathing.

COLOR BREATHING

I imagine myself breathing in my favorite color. I breathe in that color and imagine it filling up my body. (When I do this meditation, the color usually changes from day to day, so I just go with it.) Inhale your favorite color. Imagine it filling up your body. Then hold your breath for a count of five seconds.

Exhale slowly, imagining a color you hate, or just breathe out blackness.

Repeat the process.

FOUR SQUARE AND COLOR BREATHING

Try either of these meditations for five minutes. Focus on the square, or focus on the color.

If random thoughts come into your head, let them go.

It helps to shut off your phone, e-mail alerts, and put a "do not disturb" sign on your door. If you like, set an alarm so you know when your time is up.

Try it! Five minutes at a time. Slowly work your way up to twenty or thirty minutes.

Yoga

A great stress-buster (so I hear) is yoga.

Now, I'm the type of person who gets very frustrated with yoga because I'm not flexible, have never been, and never will be. So I personally hate yoga, and the frustration of it all actually makes my stress worse. But just because it doesn't work for me doesn't mean it won't work for you. Many of my patients do yoga for relaxation, and get great benefit from it.

Hatha yoga is best for this. Hatha yoga is gentle stretching and gentle poses with a focus on breathing and meditation. You should be able to find this type of yoga quite easily at a local yoga studio. Consider it yoga for beginners.

Journaling

Journaling is another effective way to let the stress go.

There are different ways to journal. You can just free-flow—whatever appears in your head you write down without thinking. Just let it all flow out.

Or you can do a gratitude journal, as I mentioned in Chapter 12: Sensational Sleep. Every day, at the end of your day, list five things you are grateful for that day. No matter how big or how small. It could be that a stranger held the door for you when your hands were full. It could be that your boss recognized your hard work. It could be that your best friend was there to listen to you vent.

Take a moment now and write down five things that you are grateful for today.

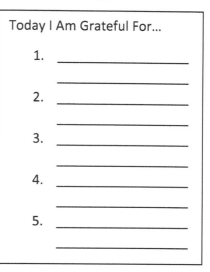

Today I Am Grateful For...

1. _____

2. _____

3. _____

4. _____

5. _____

Boxing

It may seem kind of strange that here I am telling you about meditation and yoga and gratitude journals, and the next thing I recommend is boxing.

Boxing is great vitamin R!

I told you earlier that I personally don't like yoga. I have little flexibility in my body, so I find yoga to be nothing but frustrating. But, I love boxing!

Putting on the gloves and hitting the heavy bag—man, that's a great way to shut off my brain. (I don't hit other people, just the heavy bag.) Every punch I throw has to be precise to hit the bag properly.

And, every punch I throw helps me release a bit of steam. It's empowering too. We women don't know our own strength until we do things like this! But mostly it helps me shut off my brain and let go of frustrations.

Up until I started boxing, I used to hate exercise. Sure, I would tell my patients to exercise, but I never did more than walk my dogs (I've got two Basset hounds). It was a typical case of "do what I say, not as I do."

I don't even consider boxing exercise. That's how much I love doing it. When the class is finished, I actually want to do more.

If you haven't found a form of exercise that you love doing, keep looking, and consider trying out a boxing class.

Get great sleep, take plenty of time to rest, and find some physical activity you love to fill yourself with vitamin R!

Chapter 14

You Can Feel Normal Again...Starting Now!

Congratulations! You've made it to the end of this book!

I'd like you to think of it as a new beginning. This last chapter will be the start of a new chapter in your life, where you will say good-bye to fatigue and start your new journey to Reclaim Your Energy and Feel Normal Again!

Since you're still here reading, I'll take it as a sign that you now have hope that something really can be done to fix your fatigue. You might be wondering what to do next. Here are a few thoughts for you:

1. Frankly, the quickest way for you to feel normal again is with a functional medicine doctor. Look, don't waste any more time or energy trying to figure it all out yourself. It's just too complicated and confusing. So find a functional medicine doctor, one who specializes in fatigue. Some functional medicine doctors will even work with patients from across the country using video chat or phone appointments. In fact, I know a brilliant

> To find the right functional medicine doctor for you, get your free copy of my "Consumer Awareness Guide to Functional Medicine" at www.FeelNormalAgainBook.com /SpecialBonus

functional medicine doctor who would be delighted to help you—me! (Come on, I had to get a shameless plug in at some point!)

2. Ask for a copy of your latest blood work. (If you want to have testing done, see the Resources section for specific names of tests.) Then look at your numbers. Are they in the ideal range or not? And, are there any tests that your doctor didn't run? (The specific blood tests I've mentioned earlier in this book for you to look at are: TSH, A1C (or HbA1C), B12, 25(OH) vitamin D, and ferritin.) (True story: I have a patient who lives seven hours away who sent me *all* her records—a three-inch binder full of documents! Thankfully she had it so well organized that it actually saved me a bunch of time figuring out her case!)

3. After reading about the Basic Fatigue List, do any specific areas stand out to you as a potential cause for your fatigue? Make a list of these items and tests, and then do some research to learn more about them. And if you haven't already, start making changes to your lifestyle. Come on, I know that you already know what you should do. Start today with one small step.

4. Take advantage of the Special Bonus at the end of this book and get your free copy of my Expanded Fatigue List for even more information about the underlying causes of fatigue. Make a commitment to find the underlying cause(s) of your fatigue. Sometimes it can be a real needle in a haystack. But that needle *is* there, waiting to be found! And then you can feel normal again, get your health back,

and get your life back! Remember: Find the cause. Fix the cause. Feel normal again!

5. Lastly, I want to thank you for reading this book. If you found value in it and if it has given you hope, I'd like to ask you to help me get it into the hands of other women just like you. The best and easiest way to do this is to post a review on Amazon.com. Thank you in advance for your five-star review! Also, please ask women you know if they experience fatigue. (I'll bet more do than you realize!) Tell them about this book and the proven solutions it provides. Together we can begin to cure fatigue and bring renewed health and energy to women around the globe.

Reclaim Your Energy and Feel Normal Again! Checklist

Part 1: The Hidden, Underlying Causes of Fatigue

Fatigue Factor #1: Anemia

When you have fatigue, anemia should always be checked first.

- ☐ Medical doctors check this with a CBC (complete blood count) blood test.

If any of your family members have anemia too, you should automatically be checked for:

- ☐ Celiac disease,
- ☐ non-Celiac gluten sensitivity, and
- ☐ pernicious anemia.

Fatigue Factor #2: Thyroid Problems

After checking for anemia, the thyroid should always be checked next as a possible underlying cause of your fatigue.

- ☐ Doctors test thyroid function with a TSH blood test.
- ☐ If thyroid problems run in your family, or if your medical doctor has a difficult time figuring out what dose of thyroid medication is right for you, there is a strong possibility that you actually have Hashimoto's Thyroiditis and not regular hypothyroidism. Anti-TPO and anti-TG antibody testing will confirm if this is true for you.

Fatigue Factor #3: Cortisol Imbalance

Cortisol imbalance is the most common cause of fatigue. I place it third on my list of fatigue factors since anemia and thyroid should always be checked first.

☐ Cortisol should always be tested with a saliva test, one that includes four saliva samples collected and measured throughout your average, typical day.

Fatigue Factor #4: Blood Sugar Imbalance

Along with cortisol, blood sugar imbalances are at the top of my functional medicine list as leading causes of fatigue.

☐ The blood test to see if your blood sugar is too high is the HbA1C (hemoglobin A1C) test, also called A1C for short. This test tells you the history of what your blood sugar has been doing over the last three months. This is hands down a much better test than measuring random or fasting glucose levels, which is what most doctors tend to do.

You May Be Toxic:

☐ If you know you already have high blood sugar, pre-diabetes, or even diabetes, and have been working hard on diet and exercise but are seeing little results in your blood work despite all your efforts, you may have too many toxins in your body. Oftentimes, it's only after a thorough detoxification program that blood sugar levels finally get back into balance, and you finally get your energy back.

Fatigue Factor #5: Nutrient Deficiencies

I routinely find at least one of these four nutrients as deficient in my fatigue patients:

☐ vitamin B12—can be measured with a blood test

- ☐ vitamin D—can be measured with a blood test
- ☐ magnesium—the preferred test for magnesium is an RBC magnesium (blood test)
- ☐ iron—measured with a ferritin blood test

Most women are never checked for all of these nutrients. You may want to have your doctor check.

- ☐ Don't know if your supplements are working? Try the vinegar test (or simply switch to capsule supplements only).
- ☐ If you take PPIs, safely get off them by following the recommended steps, one by one.

Fatigue Factor #6: Chronic Infections

Antibiotics are a leading cause of chronic infections.

- ☐ The easiest and best test to evaluate for hidden infections in the colon is a stool test.
- ☐ A common cause of fatigue is bacterial overgrowth in the small intestine (SIBO). The easiest and best test to evaluate for SIBO is the Lactulose Breath Test.

Fatigue Factor #7: Hidden Food Allergies & Sensitivities

IgE reactions are food allergies. IgA and IgG reactions are food sensitivities.

- ☐ You may choose to get an IgE blood test done for food allergies. Panels are commonly done for 95, 150, even 300 plus foods.

Food sensitivities can be tested with blood, but sensitivities are tricky to find.

- ☐ The best way to detect food allergies and sensitivities is to do an Elimination Diet, followed by a Food Challenge.

Fatigue Factor #8: Brain Chemical Imbalance

- ☐ Test for serotonin and dopamine: Brain Balancing—MTO Testing.
- ☐ Eat adequate protein.

Part 2: Build Your Foundation for Lasting Energy

Let Your Food Be Your Medicine

- ☐ Do the Paleo Diet.
- ☐ If you have low-grade inflammation, ditch these inflammatory foods:
  - ➢ sugar
  - ➢ carbs
  - ➢ grains
  - ➢ alcohol (okay, a little bit of red wine is allowed)
  - ➢ legumes
  - ➢ dairy
  - ➢ meat that is not organic grass fed
  - ➢ and any foods you are allergic to

Exercise to Enjoy Abundant Energy

- ☐ Do equal amounts of stretching, cardio, and resistance (weight lifting) each week.
- ☐ Exercise only until you feel energized. Too much exercise will leave you feeling drained.

Get Sensational Sleep

Identify Sleep Disturbers:

- ☐ blood sugar
- ☐ cortisol
- ☐ melatonin

Sensational Sleep Tips:

- ☐ Turn your bedroom into a dark and cozy cave.
- ☐ Establish a restful routine—follow a schedule to sleep and wake up on time.
- ☐ Get fluffy, feathery, marvelous mattresses.
- ☐ No alcohol or caffeine in the evening, and no exercise after seven at night, as these interfere with quality of sleep.

Get Rest, Relaxation, and Recreation—Vitamin R!

- ☐ Manage your stress.
- ☐ Practice deep breathing.

Meditate:

- ☐ four square breathing
- ☐ color breathing

Try:

- ☐ yoga
- ☐ journaling
- ☐ gratitude journal
- ☐ boxing *or* find some physical activity you love

And finally:

- ☐ Find a functional medicine doctor who specializes in fatigue.
- ☐ Every time you have blood work done, get a copy of the results for yourself! That way you'll know your own numbers and can start tracking them from year to year. Then if a disparity arises, you may catch what a family doctor might overlook.
- ☐ After reading about the Basic Fatigue List, do any specific areas stand out to you as a potential cause for your fatigue? Make a list of these items and tests, and then do some research to learn more about them. And if

you haven't already, start making changes to your lifestyle.

☐ Take advantage of the Special Bonus at the end of this book and get your free copy of my Expanded Fatigue List for even more information about the underlying causes of fatigue. Make a commitment to find the underlying cause(s) of your fatigue.

☐ Kindly post an enthusiastic (but realistic) review on Amazon.com. (Thank you.)

☐ Please ask women you know if they experience fatigue. Tell them about this book and the proven solutions it provides.

☐ Find the cause. Fix the cause. Feel normal again!

Resources

Functional Medicine Doctors

To find a doctor trained in functional medicine visit:

> ➤ The Institute for Functional Medicine
> www.FunctionalMedicine.org
> 1-800-228-0622
> 1-253-661-3010

Thyroid Testing

Comprehensive thyroid testing to screen for the underlying cause of low thyroid symptoms should always include:

- ✓ TSH
- ✓ Free T3
- ✓ Free T4
- ✓ Total T3
- ✓ Total T4
- ✓ Anti-TPO (Thyroperoxidase) antibodies
- ✓ Anti-TG (Thyroglobulin) antibodies
- ✓ Reverse T3

Most, if not all, of these tests can be performed through any standard medical laboratory.

Cortisol Testing (Functional Adrenal Stress Profile)

- ➢ BioHealth Laboratory—(#201—Functional Adrenal Stress Profile, or #205—Functional Adrenal Stress Profile Plus V)
  www.BioHealthLab.com
  1-800-570-2000
  1-307-426-5060

- ➢ DiagnosTechs—(Adrenal Stress Index)
  www.DiagnosTechs.com
  1-800-878-3787
  1-425-251-0596

Vitamin D Testing

Most standard labs offer vitamin D testing. But these labs offer the vitamin D finger prick test:

- ➢ Rocky Mountain Analytical Lab
  www.RMALab.com
  1-403-241-4500

- ➢ ZRT Laboratory
  www.ZRTLab.com
  1-866-600-1636

Breath Test for SIBO (Small Intestinal Bacteria Overgrowth)

- ➢ Commonwealth Laboratories—(Small Intestinal Bacteria Overgrowth (SIBO) Breath Test)
  www.HydrogenBreathTesting.com
  1-800-292-9019
  1-781-659-0704

Stool Testing for Hidden Infections

> ➢ BioHealth Laboratory—(#401H test—GI Pathogen Screen with H. pylori Antigen)
> www.BioHealthLab.com
> 1-800-570-2000
> 1-307-426-5060

> ➢ Doctor's Data—(Comprehensive Stool Analysis with Parasitology x 3)
> www.DoctorsData.com
> 1-800-323-2784

> ➢ Metametrix Clinical Laboratory—(GI Effects Comprehensive Stool Profile)
> www.Metametrix.com
> 1-800-221-4640
> 1-770-446-5483

Food Allergy Testing: Blood Testing

These labs offer food allergy/sensitivity testing for IgE, IgA, and IgG antibodies:

> ➢ Rocky Mountain Analytical Lab
> www.RMALab.com
> 1-403-241-4500

> ➢ US BioTek Laboratories
> www.USBioTek.com
> 1-877-318-8728
> 1-206-365-1256

Brain Balancing—MTO (Monoamine Transporter Optimization) Testing

To find a doctor trained in MTO testing, ask for a doctor near you who has specifically been trained in the Mind Mapping Program:

> ➤ The Kalish Institute
> www.KalishWellness.com
> 1-800-616-7708

Pelvic Floor Rehabilitation

To find a physiotherapist who has specialized training in pelvic floor rehabilitation, you will have to do some research on your own. First, look for one specialized in women's health. Then, interview them. Ask about their training and experience specifically with pelvic floor rehabilitation. Ask if they exclusively use manual therapy methods, or if they also use biofeedback or electrical stimulation. The physiotherapist you want will *only* rely on manual therapy. Here are two Web sites where you can search for physiotherapists:

> ➤ www.Physiotherapy.ca

> ➤ www.OPA.on.ca

Sleep Hygiene

Room darkening window coverings that are easy to install:

> ➤ www.BlackoutEZ.com

Melatonin Testing

➤ BioHealth Laboratory—(#254—Melatonin)
www.BioHealthLab.com
1-800-570-2000
1-307-426-5060

Special Bonus

Bonus #1

Get your free copy of my Expanded Fatigue List, including fatigue causes ("fatigue factors") #9 to #14.

Bonus #2

Get your free copy of my "Consumer Awareness Guide to Functional Medicine." In this guide you'll discover how to avoid three common functional medicine rip-offs, five misconceptions about functional medicine, eight questions to ask before you book your first appointment with a functional medicine doctor, and four mistakes to avoid when choosing your functional medicine doctor.

Bonus #3

Get your free copy of "Six Truths You Need to Hear about Natural Treatments for Fatigue... Like It or Not."

Get immediate access to these reports by going to www.ReclaimYourEnergyBook.com/SpecialBonus

Bibliography

Books:

Why Do I Still Have Thyroid Symptoms? When My Lab Tests Are Normal
Datis Kharrazian
http://www.amazon.ca/Still-Thyroid-Symptoms-Tests-Normal/dp/0985690402

Migraine Headaches, Hypothyroidism, and Fibromyalgia: Assessments and Therapeutic Approaches Using Integrative Chiropractic, Naturopathic, Osteopathic, and Functional Medicine
Alex Vasquez
http://www.amazon.ca/Migraine-Headaches-Hypothyroidism-Fibromyalgia-Chiropractic/dp/1468123734/ref=sr_1_3?s=books&ie=UTF8&qid=1398353208&sr=1-3

Functional Immunology and Nutritional Immunomodulation: Presentation Slides Part 1: Introduction to the Use of Nutrition and Functional Medicine in The Prevention and Treatment of Chronic Inflammation, Allergy, Autoimmunity...and the new FIND SEX Acronym
Alex Vasquez
http://www.amazon.ca/Functional-Immunology-Nutritional-Immunomodulation-Presentation/dp/1477603859/ref=sr_1_12?s=books&ie=UTF8&qid=1398353208&sr=1-12

A New IBS Solution: Bacteria—The Missing Link in Treating Irritable Bowel Syndrome
Mark Pimentel
http://www.amazon.ca/New-IBS-Solution-Bacteria-The-Irritable/dp/0977435601

Nutritional Medicine
Alan Gaby
http://www.amazon.com/Nutritional-Medicine-Alan-Gaby/dp/B005ERQLS4

Textbook of Functional Medicine
Sidney MacDonald Baker (author), Peter Bennett (author), & 8 more
http://www.amazon.com/Textbook-Functional-Medicine-Sidney-MacDonald/dp/0977371301

The Kalish Method: Healing the Body, Mapping the Mind
Daniel Kalish
http://www.amazon.ca/The-Kalish-Method-Healing-Mapping/dp/1477612726

The Paleo Diet Revised: Lose Weight and Get Healthy by Eating the Foods You Were Designed to Eat
Loren Cordain
http://www.amazon.com/The-Paleo-Diet-Revised-Designed/dp/0470913029

The Plan: Eliminate the Surprising "Healthy" Foods That Are Making You Fat--and Lose Weight Fast
Lyn-Genet Recitas
http://www.amazon.com/dp/1455515485/ref=as_li_tf_til?tag=ww wlyngenetco-
20&camp=14573&creative=327641&linkCode=as1&creativeASI N=1455515485&adid=19Y4K13TJQG1S0XFFRZ6&&ref-refURL=http%3A%2F%2Frcm.amazon.com%2Fe%2Fcm%3Ft%3 Dwwwlyngenetco-
20%26o%3D1%26p%3D8%26l%3Das1%26asins%3D145551548 5%26ref%3Dtf_til%26fc1%3D000000%26IS2%3D1%26lt1%3D_ blank%26m%3Damazon%26lc1%3D0000FF%26bc1%3D000000 %26bg1%3DFFFFFF%26f%3Difr

Clinical Nutrition: A Functional Approach
http://www.amazon.ca/Clinical-Nutrition-A-Functional-Approach/dp/0962485918

Seminars:

Functional Endocrinology, 2003. Datis Kharrazian, DC, DHSc, MS, MNeuroSci, FAACP, FACFN, DACNB, DABCN, DIBAK, CNS.

Mastering the Thyroid, 2009. Datis Kharrazian, DC, DHSc, MS, MNeuroSci, FAACP, FACFN, DACNB, DABCN, DIBAK, CNS.

Clinical Nutrition: How dietary habits drive diseases throughout the lifecycle & key nutritional interventions, 2011. David Seaman, DC, MS, DACBN.

The Kalish Method Mentorship, 2012.
http://kalishinstitute.com/mentorship/

Functional & Nutritional Immunology, 2012. Alex Vasquez, DC, ND, DO.

Vitamin D Disease Prevention Symposium, 2012. Robert P. Heaney, MD; Carole A. Baggerly; Marc Sorenson, EdD.

Mind Mapping: The Next Generation of Amino Acid Therapy, 2012 – 2013. Dr. Dan Kalish, DC.

The Gluten Summit, 2013. Dr. Tom O'Bryan, DC. http://theglutensummit.com/

> ➤ Before Marsh III: Why the Early Stages of Celiac Disease Must be Taken Seriously
> Michael Marsh, MD, DSc, FRCP

> ➤ Eliminating Gluten as the 1st Step in Preventing Brain Conditions
> David Perlmutter, MD, FACN, ABIHM

> ➤ Why Creating the Healthiest Intestinal Environment Possible Can Arrest Your Vulnerability to the #3 Cause of Getting Sick and Dying
> Alessio Fasano, MD

> ➤ Properly Testing for Gluten Sensitivity and Why Current Methods Fail
> Aristo Vojdani, PhD, MSc, MT

> ➤ A "Functional Approach" to Lifestyle Can Transform Your Body
> Mark Hyman, MD

> ➤ The Reality of Non-Celiac Gluten Sensitivity and Its Many Manifestations
> Umberto Volta, MD

➤ Are You Developing an Autoimmune Disease Years Before Symptoms?
Prof. Yehuda Shoenfeld, MD, FRCP

Health Fusion 2013—The Integrative Treatment of Chronic Inflammatory Conditions. The Canadian Association of Naturopathic Doctors

The Gastrointestinal Masterclass, 2014. Jason Hawrelak, ND, BNat (Hons), PhD.

SIBO Symposium, 2014. http://sibosymposium.com/

About the Author

Dr. Carri Drzyzga is known internationally as The Functional Medicine Doc. She is committed to helping patients find the root cause of their health problems and fix the cause with natural treatments so they can feel normal again.

Her last name is pronounced "**Driz**-ga" (it is Polish), but everyone simply calls her Dr. Carri.

She has been in private practice since 1996, and is founder of Functional Medicine Ontario in Ottawa, Ontario.

Dr. Carri holds two doctoral degrees—Chiropractic and Naturopathic Medicine. Additionally, she has training in Functional Medicine and The Kalish Method, and is a Certified Gluten Practitioner. Always an avid learner, Dr. Carri has obtained a level of expertise in her profession that no other doctor in Canada has achieved to date.

Dr. Carri speaks and gives interviews on such topics as natural treatments for fatigue, chronic pain, hypothyroidism, and immune and digestive health. She has enjoyed being a featured guest on The New RO and CTV news channels and being a featured speaker at The Eastern Ontario Chiropractic Society.

Dr. Carri has been married for eighteen years to her husband Benoît, who is also a chiropractor. They have two rescued Basset hounds, Bailey and Sammi, who couldn't be chiropractors because of their lack of opposable thumbs and propensity for slobbering on patients. Carri and Ben like to travel, hike, and just spend time together.

For more resources and information on Dr. Carri, visit:

➢ www.DrCarri.com

➢ www.Facebook.com/DrCarri

➢ www.FunctionalMedicineOntario.com

➢ www.ReclaimYourEnergyBook.com

➢ www.DrCarri.TV